Diagnosis: Lupus

The Intimate Journal of a Lupus Patient

Marilyn Celeste Morris

PublishAmerica
Baltimore

First printing

ISBN: 1-4137-6789-3
PUBLISHED BY
PUBLISHAMERICA, LLLP.
www.publishamerica.com
Baltimore

Printed in the United States of America

Acknowledgements

I would like to thank The Lupus Foundation of America for providing timely information to thousands of those seeking answers to this devastating disease;

The North Texas Chapter of the LFA, particularly its board members, for donating their time and expertise to raise lupus awareness and treatment in our communities;

The vice president of the North Texas Chapter of the LFA, Paula Frazier; and Stephanie Lanier, Secretary—thanks for your hard work setting up seminars, presentations to civic groups, making the thousands of telephone calls, sending emails necessary for a viable and active presence in this area...

The co-facilitators of The Fort Worth Lupus Support Group, Lee Ann Dailey, Janice Hawbaker and Kathy DiSalvo, for leading the meetings in my absence (and for keeping the meeting on track when I suffer a lupus lapse);

And to all the members of the lupus support groups, past, present and future, for your courage in sharing your frustrations, pain and recovery with us—a room full of strangers when you entered, but a network of friends when you leave.

Thanks also to my dear friends who bore with me in the dark days before diagnosis, too numerous to name, who propped me up when I felt I couldn't go on any more, and applied a swift kick to my posterior when needed; most of them are members of the Al-Anon Family Group, who, by example, taught me to trust God and keep walking...

To all my physicians, who did the best they could at the time, in attempting to diagnose and treat this stubborn, cynical patient—my belated apologies for having impugned your integrity, knowledge and skills (and at times, questioning your ancestry!)

To all my counselors, those underpaid, dedicated souls, who "stitched me up" whenever I came unraveled.

And to my family—son, Woody, daughters, Terri and Lauri, who all feared they would lose their mother to the ravages of this disease; my brothers, Gary and Robert.

And to my parents—R.M. and Frances Morris.

Just where do you suppose I got my strength?

Foreword

ENTRIES FROM MY JOURNAL DETAIL MY PERSONAL STRUGGLE for diagnosis and treatment of systemic lupus erythematosus (lupus) from the first symptoms in 1982, diagnosis in 1988, to my current, thank God, state of remission. Please note that I have changed the names of my doctors, hospitals, and other data to protect their identities.

My purpose is to inform, in non-clinical language, newly-diagnosed, yet-to-be diagnosed patients and their families; give them courage to continue seeking a diagnosis in the face of frustration and feelings of despair; and offer hope, even when conditions seem hopeless.

By relating my innermost thoughts and feelings, I hope readers will come to realize they are not alone in their frustration, depression, job losses and subsequent loss of income, battles with an alphabet soup of public assistance services, Social Security disability; food stamps and weight gain. Nobody wants the inevitable weight gain and subsequent loss of self-esteem that comes with the taking of steroids, but "you pays your money and you takes your choice." Personally, I'd rather be twenty pounds over my ideal weight, walking around, than skinny in my coffin.

Questions such as "How did I get this disease? Will my children also get it? Why doesn't my doctor tell me anything except 'You've got lupus; take this medicine and come back in three months'? will be addressed, along with many others.

Although many journal entries detail my struggles with clinical depression, job losses, loss of income and other dire consequences of this disease, my intent is not to linger there, but to press on toward remission, recovery and acceptance.

As many new members of our local lupus support groups sigh in relief upon finding us, "I thought I was the only person in the world who felt this way," so will readers discover they are truly not alone in their thinking and their feelings.

While I compiled these entries from the perspective of a "recovered" lupus patient, I am also aware that lupus may rear its ugly head at any moment, bringing me back to the rounds of physicians, medications, and even hospitalization. This is the life persons with chronic diseases must lead, and their choices are either to feel sorry for themselves and burrow into a sinkhole of despair, or live life as it comes, one day at a time, the best way possible.

I have known persons who have lost the battle and I certainly want to live a long and healthy life.

I also know that tomorrow, my life may be ended in a freak accident.

My choice is, "I'm not going to stop living just so I can live."

Introduction
May 2002

"ARE YOU SURE YOU HAVE LUPUS?" MY NEWEST DOCTOR ASKED as he entered the exam room, my lab tests from the week before in his hands.

"Yes. I was diagnosed in October 1988," I replied. "Why? What do the tests show?"

"Well, they show no sign of lupus. No ANA, sed rate is normal, no RA factor…"

"Great!" I burbled. "Suppose I'm in remission?"

"Or maybe you never really had lupus." He shrugged.

For one crazy, hopeful moment, I actually thought: *Maybe he's right. Maybe I didn't really have lupus, after all.*

Then my thoughts flooded to the three years of constant joint pain, lab tests, five doctors telling me it was either "All in my head" or "Just rheumatoid arthritis" all the while being told not enough symptoms were showing in the blood work.

NEVER REALLY HAD LUPUS? I wanted to shout: Then what was all the lung infection, the hair loss, the treatments with

Cytoxan, Imuran, prednisone; the difficulty walking when vasculitis caused foot drop in both feet and I fell down a lot? Frustration mounted on frustration as the disease progressed.

NEVER REALLY HAD LUPUS? Then what was with my red, swollen joints, causing one rheumatologist to rhapsodize, "What beautiful swollen knees!" When I couldn't wear rings, watches or bracelets because of the intense pain and swelling? When even my collarbones hurt?

NEVER REALLY HAD LUPUS? Then what was all the bouncing from job to job, being fired or quitting due to sheer physical exhaustion, or finding it impossible to concentrate on the task at hand?

NEVER REALLY HAD LUPUS? Then why did I break out in a fiery rash after being in the sun? What was the point in hauling my body out of bed at 5:30 a.m., climbing painfully into a tub or hot water, eating breakfast so I could swallow my handful of meds (that didn't seem to be doing much good) so I could get dressed and have my butt in a chair at my office-du-jour by 8:00 a.m.?

NEVER REALLY HAD LUPUS? Then what was all the memory loss about? What words escaped me at just the right time to embarrass me so that I could only shrug and murmur, "Lupus lapse" much as Richard Fish on *Ally McBeal* shrugged, "Bygones."

Rather than lash out at this newest, most optimistic young doctor, I merely smiled and shrugged, "Yes, I really did have lupus."

I wish I could tell you that my disease came on suddenly, that I went to the doctor, was diagnosed and treated immediately, and everybody lived happily ever after.

Unfortunately, that didn't happen. Nor does it happen with the majority of lupus patients; at least with those I've known. After three years full of pain, doubt, fear, and anger, and after changing doctors, both primary care physicians and rheumatologists, *five* times, I was at last diagnosed with SLE.

And my treatment took a very long time, and brought with it, not the expected relief of pain, doubt, fear and anger, but *Four*

(Other) Horsemen of This Disease: Weight gain, high blood pressure, diabetes, and vasculitis. I must also add clinical depression, job loss, loss of income, foreclosure, lining up for food stamps, medicines and other Public Assistance services. I was truly humbled when I picked up my handicapped parking tag, food stamps and vouchers. I was infuriated by low-level clerks who used their positions of power to assert their superiority over me, verbally slapping my wrists, and at one point, one even shaking her finger at me, yet I had to submit in order to get whatever assistance they could offer.

I had a meltdown in my parish priest's office, confessing that I needed financial help; I had a true gasping-for-air, snot-slinging hissy fit in the college library after I was told I might not be able to complete my schooling. And all this time, I tried to reassure my family and friends that I would not, could not, leave this crappy world via my own hand, even though I admitted, however, I *would* just like to *lie down and die*.

That's what this disease did *to* me.

This is what this disease did *for* me.

I learned there is a God, and I'm not Him/Her.

I learned that God loves me as much as He loves you.

I learned I'm not perfect, never have been, never will be, and that's okay.

I learned that this disease is not a punishment for "sins."

I learned how to ask for help.

I learned how to be grateful for and accept that help.

I learned that things are merely objects, that money is simply a means to an end, and not the be-all and end-all of life.

I learned the difference between *needs* and *wants*.

I learned to surrender, to "Let go and let God."

I learned that expectations are only premeditated resentments.

I learned not to discount the message because of the messenger.

If all of the above sounds vaguely familiar to those of you who are members of a 12-Step Recovery group, you are correct. I make no secret of the fact that I am a grateful member of the

9

Al-Anon Family Group, and lest anyone fear I am breaking my anonymity, my last name is not the same as my children's or my ex-husband's, since I wisely had my maiden name restored upon my divorce.

When I mention friends' names, some are members of the fellowship, some are not. I have, however, changed the names of the doctors and institutions, simply because I believe it serves no purpose to impugn their reputations. I also know today that they did the best they could with the information available at the time. They're not perfect, and they certainly aren't gods.

When I write of my parents' shortcomings, I am not "parent-bashing" or playing "Let's blame Mom and Dad." My parents weren't perfect, any more than my doctors were perfect; they also did the best they could during my childhood and in trying to cope with their feelings about my illness.

I give thanks daily that I was already a member of the Al-Anon Family Group and the Episcopal Church before the onset of symptoms of SLE. While working with my sponsor, while studying to be a Stephen Minister, and while literally crying on my dear friends' shoulders, I was sustained by their love and caring support. By holding me in their arms, keeping me in their prayers, and yes, by giving me swift kicks to the posterior, these people kept me alive. To this day, I don't know how they managed to listen to my constant crying, complaints, and self-doubts, much less stand stoically as they heard me rage at God, myself and the entire universe for whatever was going wrong in my life.

Because of them, I am alive. Today.

And I know today that is all we have—this day. This moment.

I hope my experiences inform you, strengthen you, and give you hope.

First, Some Facts...

Some symptoms of lupus:

Do you have/ever had/been told you have:

Achy, painful and/or swollen joints for more than three months;

Fingers and/or toes becoming pale, numb or uncomfortable in the cold;

Sores in the mouth for more than two weeks;

Been told you have a low blood count, anemia, low white cell count or a low platelet count;

Ever had a prominent redness or color change in the shape of a butterfly across the bridge of your nose and cheeks;

An unexplained fever over 100 degrees for more than a few days;

A sensitivity to the sun where the skin breaks out after being in the sun (not a sunburn);

Had chest pain with breathing for more than a few days (pleurisy);

Been told you had protein in your urine;

Experienced persistent, extreme fatigue and weakness for days or weeks at a time even after 6-8 hours of restful nighttime sleep.

If you have 3 or more symptoms, you should see your doctor.

According to the Lupus Foundation of America, lupus is more common than leukemia, Hodgkin's disease, muscular dystrophy, Cystic fibrosis and multiple sclerosis. And yet, the average person rarely knows about lupus and is generally misinformed, vaguely believing it to be "kind of like arthritis, isn't it?" While my symptoms first presented themselves as "kind of like arthritis," and I was thus diagnosed and treated for two years for RA, other symptoms soon presented themselves, until, after three emotionally charged and pain-filled years from the onset of symptoms, laboratory tests confirmed the presence of SLE, or systemic lupus erythematosus.

There are two distinct types of lupus. One is discoid lupus, where the skin shows large "splotches" or red rashes in clusters, mostly on the face, across the cheeks and the bridge of the nose, creating a "wolf-like" mask. One can have discoid lupus and systemic lupus at the same time; generally, those who suffer with the discoid form of lupus do not develop the systemic form.

The second is systemic lupus; that is, it is throughout the body. It has been classified as "an autoimmune disease."

Lupus has nothing to do with AIDS, I must point out. I like the 'short,' understandable description of what lupus is: Think of the body as a fort, like in the Wild West days. Every now and then, Indians would attack the fort, and the soldiers inside the fort (white blood cells) would repel the Indians (the infection). Then the fort (body) would settle down and go back to its usual routine, until the next Indian attack

Only with lupus, there are no Indians. The soldiers inside the fort are ever ready for an attack, but the Indians don't arrive, so the soldiers (stressed) turn on each other, fighting among themselves, eventually destroying the fort itself: lungs, kidneys, central nervous system, etc.

As of this printing, there is no cure, but it is treatable.

Words to the Newly Diagnosed, Undiagnosed and Their Families....

Actually, one word: Hope. There *is* hope. Despite the pain, the despair, the uncertainty, and the fatigue—there is a light at the end of the tunnel. While listening to new members of our local lupus support group, I hear their fear.

"I thought I was the only person in the world who felt this way."

"Did your doctor tell you it was all in your head?"

"Did your doctor tell you it was 'just' rheumatoid arthritis?"

"My family does not understand what I'm going through. After all, I don't look sick."

"How can you work when you have lupus?"

"How can I get Social Security disability? They keep denying my claim."

"My company fired me after I took disability. Is this legal?"

"How can I find work when I'm so sick?"

"How do you manage the pain?"

"What does cortisone do to your body?"

"Why isn't the medication my doctor prescribed for me doing me any good? I still hurt."

"Why doesn't my doctor tell me more about lupus? All he said was, 'You have lupus. Take this medicine and come back in three months.'"

"My doctor won't talk to me when I call his office. His office staff tells me he's busy, or he can't talk to me, and they won't answer my questions. What should I do?"

"How do I answer people's questions when I tell them I have lupus?"

And, the topper: "People tell me, 'You don't look sick. You look too healthy to be sick.'"

And their unspoken questions, as much as those uttered: Will I die from this? How long will I be sick? Will I get worse? What about kidney involvement? Seizures? Why did I get this disease? Will my children also get it?

Difficult questions, indeed.

I disagree with the perception that you must have not lived a good, clean life, or you wouldn't have developed cancer, diabetes—or SLE. If anything, my life had been "squeaky-clean" up to age 20, when I married for the first time.

I do believe, however, with the perception that stress plays a major role in illness' development, and, Lord knows, I had enough stress in my life.

And so does everyone.

Stress, good or bad (marriage, children being born, promotions, are all stressors) has an effect on one's mind and body. By the time I reached age 44, I had had several major stressors, and I reacted the way I always had—chin up, swallowed my hurt and anger, and got on with it.

Most of us Lupans have had a great deal of stress in our lives. We are, after all, overachievers. We take on more than the ordinary person. We are perfectionists. We work too hard, don't know how to play, and don't rest when we should. And that's *before* we get lupus. So it's extremely difficult to "take it easy" when diagnosed with this disease.

So with my stress, I didn't take the time to grieve over my divorces, to rage aloud at the injustices in my life.

I simmered. And my body, seeking an outlet for such stress buildup, rebelled. Like volcanoes, fires erupted in my joints, cartilage and ligaments. My emotional pain had been crying out for attention.

It was physical pain that got my attention.

What my personal journey through this darkness has taught me is this: The disease is worst at the beginning—before diagnosis and treatment.

As in my case, I was diagnosed in October 1988 and hospitalized with a raging case of pleuritis in March 1989. This was preceded, of course, by at least three years of constant searching for a diagnosis, going from doctor to doctor, bouncing from job to job as my energy level waned and deteriorated, and dealing with an alphabet soup of medical institutions, insurance companies, mental health and rehabilitation facilities. And then, despite the aggressive treatment, my body succumbed at last.

But back to the beginning statement…It's worse in the beginning.

Once the lab tests come back with a positive for SLE, and treatment is begun, you can get better. I promise. You might also get worse before you get better. I promise that, too. But you will get to the point where the pain abates, anxiety lessens, mobility is restored and confidence in living a full life returns.

It will take time, medications, and dedication on your part to adhere to the treatment plan your physician has outlined for you (keeping in mind "You must become your own best physician") and determination to defeat the beast that has taken up residence in your body.

A support system is essential. Family, friends, church—learn to lean on them for a change. I know, I know, we have always been the ones to comfort, rather than be comforted. To give, rather than receive, care, compassion and chicken soup to those in need.

This is your turn.

Embarrassed? It's nothing you did or didn't do. You don't blame your son's Sunday school teacher for having cancer, do you? It happens. Through no fault of his/hers.

Still, I questioned: "Why me? Why now?"

Because, that's why, my mother/myself said.

I did cry a lot when the lupus was at its worst. I wanted the pain to end; although I didn't want to commit suicide, there were times when I sincerely wanted to just lie down and die.

While looking back on my journals for use in writing this book, I was struck by what seemed at first as an inordinate amount of "whining." But, by golly, I needed to whine. Indeed, I not only "whined," I complained. I ranted. Frustrated beyond belief, I lashed out at those around me. And I railed against God Himself.

Yet somehow, I was sustained through this challenging time in my life. I attained an unexpected spiritual growth in the face of this adversity. Years ago, I would have gagged on the "goody two-shoes" phrases, believing there was noting "spiritual" about having any illness. God was against me, if He existed at all, and certainly, I didn't feel "noble" about suffering with this dammed disease.

I took heart from one of the many books I read where one of the chapters was titled, "Dying Is the Easy Part." I knew it would be easier to die than to stand up and fight this disease. I've never been known to take the easy way out, however. So I allowed myself to cry.

My doctor said, "You've got a right to sing the blues," and sing them I did.

I had the determination to beat this disease, but I needed help —beyond that of modern medicine.

"Life is Difficult" M. Scott Peck wrote in *The Road Less Traveled.*

Nobody had ever told me that before. Any little annoyance, inconvenience, or major lifestyle change caused me to rebel. "It's not fair. Life isn't supposed to be like this. Bad things happen to other people, but not to me. I've been good."

Rabbi Harold Kushner wrote pretty much the same thing in his landmark book: *When Bad Things Happen to Good People* and the truth finally dawned on me: *Life happens.*

Laughter is essential. Norman Cousins, in his book, *Anatomy of an Illness*, tells how he rented a hotel room, a projector and old Marx Brothers movies, and laughed his way out of the pain. A good 30 minutes of laughter enabled him to sleep where he could not before.

I began keeping a journal. After all, I had whined to my family and friends enough. I needed to vent. I needed to feel sorry for myself even while I presented a brave front to the world. This journal led me to a special kind of healing. I began a spiritual and physical journey, realizing one cannot be undertaken without the other.

I would someday use these entries for my story about lupus, I thought. But when every other journal entry contained references to laments of financial worries, fear and insecurities. I wondered, "Who would want to wade through all these recitations of woe? Reading about chronic illness is not a favorite choice, anyway; if a person has lupus, isn't it enough to just read the facts and go on?"

No, it isn't, in my humble opinion. I could read all the statistics in the world and still not feel like anyone understands how I feel—what's actually going on inside me, emotionally, as well as dry numbers on a sed rate scale. More than anything else, I believe, I wanted people to know that the pain I was experiencing encompassed more than every joint/connective tissue/vital organ of my body. That pain influenced every area of my life...physical, mental, emotional and spiritual.

I wanted people to know that I was, indeed, legitimately

suffering from the slings and arrows of outrageous fortune, even though I "looked wonderful."

Lupus patients truly don't "look sick." Unlike cancer, lupus does not leave its victims looking pale, gaunt, and emaciated. We appear in radiant good health, while lupus may be silently destroying our kidneys. We look—ahem—overfed, overweight— pumped up on steroids, our faces get rounder and rounder; our trunks also bloom while the limbs remain the same. An odd appearance, to say the least, and one that is not welcomed by its hosts, prompting remarks such as "How can you be so sick when you look so—uh—(Say it—dammit! Fat!) healthy."

We generally have no visible disabilities, either, like Parkinson's patients. There are usually no tremors, no speech difficulties, and no problems with ambulating. Certain forms of lupus, of course, can lead to seizures, psychoses, and other neurological defects, but generally, we appear healthy.

Treatment for lupus is non-dramatic, as a cancer's chemotherapy. Yes, we take pills. Lots of pills. Generally, we are not forced into being "hooked up to tubes" intravenously. But the meds also give us hair loss, violent rashes and scars on our fragile skin, and our eyes must be protected from the sunlight.

Many of us work, at least part-time, as our illness allows. Sometimes we go into remission, for days, weeks, months, years, and we rejoice in those times. But when lupus bites into us, wearing us down with fatigue, pain, arthritic-like hands, swollen knees, malfunctioning kidneys or other organs, and neurological misfires, we are truly, once again, very sick.

Even if we still look in the best of health.

Some days you're the bug, some days you're the windshield.

My Search Begins

VICTIM: A living being used as a sacrifice in a religious ceremony, a person or thing destroyed or hurt in the pursuit of some object; one injured or killed by some misfortune or calamity; a sufferer from mental or physical disease; a dupe.

SUFFER: To feel (up-bear) what is painful, disagreeable or distressing; endure with pain or distress; as to suffer a wrong; to feel or bear upward, as to suffer pain; to be affected by, exercise, undergo; to allow; permit; To experience pain, loss, distress. Endure, support, tolerate.

I searched for a label to pin on my puzzling symptoms:

The inability to type all day at a word processor. The inability to sit, stand and walk for eight hours in a day without extreme fatigue. The inability to understand and implement simple verbal instructions due to a puzzling and devastating "fog" that enveloped my cognitive functions at crucial moments. And, if it hadn't been so critical to my job performance, the temporary loss of verbal ability resulting in garbled and stuttering answers to my supervisors' questions. Needless to say, I was "let go" several times.

Some diseases begin so dramatically, so definitively, that there is no question in any physician's mind as to the diagnosis. A lump in the breast calls for immediate biopsy and lab tests. A sudden sharp pain in the chin sends the patient to the emergency room where high-tech equipment confirms the presence of heart disease.

Not so with lupus. This disease presents itself with such a myriad of symptoms that its sufferers begin to doubt their sanity. Pain, stiffness in the joints surely must mean arthritis—or, as several of my former physicians dismissed it casually, after all, at your age, just learn to live with it.

Sudden and dramatic weight loss, a boon to any woman struggling with her self-image ("Well, I see you've lost a lot of weight recently. Good for you; keep it up.") Instead of an alarm that something is wrong. Other symptoms, such as extreme fatigue cause even the patient to question herself. "Tired? How can I be so tired that I just want to lie down and not even move? I must be lazy. No, I really have to nap before dinner...*what is wrong with me?*"

Weeks, even months pass, with no improvement. Symptoms

worsen. After the family physician, his knowledge exhausted, and extensive lab tests reveal nothing unusual, the patient is labeled a hypochondriac. There is *really nothing wrong*, she is told.

But the pain makes believing this difficult. While seated on a stool in the shower, unable to stand the woman notices in horror that large clumps of hair are flowing down the drain. When she manages to pull herself together for some social event, she teeters on the brink of exhaustion only to be scolded on the way home by her husband/companion/family.

"I don't understand how you can be tired all the time. The doctor says there's nothing wrong, with all the expensive lab tests..." leaving the rest of the sentence unspoken. "It's all in your mind."

After a time, after months and years of unrelenting, unforgiving, baffling, excruciating, agonizing, subtle, intense, bouts of fatigue arid other odd symptoms, resignation sets in. If relationships are good to begin with, the family considers the patient somewhat "strange," and tolerates her odd behavior pattern with dark humor, somewhat like keeping a crazy maiden aunt locked in the attic. Already strained marriages or other relationships, on the other hand, crack wide open and the partner's "psychosomatic illnesses" provide a good excuse for leaving the marriage or severing the relationship.

Even within the community of family or friends, an undiagnosed lupus patient is left to cope as best she can—feeling useless, burdensome to others, sometimes to the point of suicide.

After all, nobody can believe that this person who shows no obvious physical signs of disease—is indeed, ill—in fact, she is "glowing with good health," apparently, and gaining weight, to boot. "How can you be sick when you look so—well?" becomes a constant refrain. (Meaning, of course, "How can you be sick when you're so—fat?")

The weight gain, moon face, trunk swollen with an extra twenty or thirty pounds, on average comes after massive doses of Prednisone quells the initial pain of the disease but the toll it takes on one's body, and emotions, begins to show. A young woman who had been a model in her pre-lupus days, gains one hundred pounds, breaks a hip through necrosis, loses her marvelous long black hair, can't find work due to the pain involved in simple movements, moves back to her parents' house, and she becomes suicidal. There is nothing left before her except more pain, more days full of idleness, seeing her swollen body day after day negating the happy, vivacious creature she was a few short months earlier.

I was a little older than the typical lupus patient, but I fit the other profile. Lupus patients (or, Lupans) are busy people, working and playing 25 hours a day. They don't know when to quit; they are perfectionists and they have an unquenchable interest in nearly everything.

Their pain threshold is astonishing; I was typical in the way I ignored the first symptoms until they became almost unbearable. Likewise, the tolerance for stress. My motto was, "What stress?" and I was really quite unaware of the tremendous amounts of stress I had been under during most of my life, particularly the last few years. And that's good stress, as well as bad stress.

When I told people that I had Lupus, I got one of several reactions: "What's that?" or, "Lupus? Don't people die from that?" One callous person asked, "Is it fatal?" and I shot back with, "Yes. Of course. Life is fatal."

Bless my friends' hearts; they understood when I had to cancel a social event at the last minute, because I was "crashing" where I had been "fine" a few moments earlier.

How did this disease come to reside in me?

Heredity had a large part in my illness: My mother's mother, Emily Richardson, was half Native American; my mother was born in Sels, Arizona, and spent the first three years of her life on the Indian Reservation there. On my father's side, I claim a great-great-grandmother, Pernicia Blackwell, who had some Seminole Indian background. (North American Indians and African-Americans are prime targets of lupus.)

Besides the ordinary childhood diseases, chickenpox at age 6, mumps at the age of 12, and chronic bronchitis until I "outgrew it" at age 14, I contracted diphtheria in infancy. One of my first memories—if not my very first memory—is of lying on a bed with warm steam rising to the top of a makeshift "tent" of sheets as I struggled for every breath. This memory surfaced dramatically and unexpectedly when at the ripe old age of 60, I arrived at the emergency room one evening suffering a full-blown asthma attack and the well-meaning nurse thrust a steaming mask at my face; I shot up off the gurney in a visceral, knee-jerk reaction, striking at her hand in an infantile way. She backed off while I sat, perplexed at my response, and then she offered me a mouth tube, which I gladly accepted.

I was born right before WWII to a young PFC and his teenage wife, in Alpine, Texas. A short time later, I was whisked into the nomadic life of a military brat, as I accompanied my parents all over the world. Exciting, yes, but stressful, too. Every few years I would have to reinvent myself as I entered yet another school as "the new kid in class." "My" military career ended when my father retired in 1958.

And that same year I got married. And the same year I had my first child—a two pound fourteen ounce boy we had to leave in the hospital until he gained up to five pounds. And we had no insurance, as my husband was still a college student. And my parents moved to California. We moved to California, and then we had another baby, a girl, and moved to Lubbock, Texas. There, I developed a mysterious illness that put me in the hospital for various tests; I was so weak and fatigued I could barely summon the strength to get out of bed each morning. It was determined, after the fact, that I had contracted a case of mononucleosis, which went untreated, and then had invaded my liver, causing a raging case of hepatitis. The prescription was complete bed rest for six weeks and B12 shots daily. Immediately upon my recovery, we moved to San Antonio, Texas, where in 1968 we gave our marriage a mercy killing. I moved again with my children to Fort Worth to be closer to my own parents. Two years later, I married again.

As we say now, "We all got married." My husband had

custody of his 3-year-old girl who needed a mommy; I had two children who needed a daddy, sooooo...

And twelve years after that, another divorce. This marriage was ripped apart by alcoholism and infidelity and my stress level escalated to the point where I was always on edge, on guard, and developed "female problems" which required attention; the end result was a sudden and unexpected hysterectomy.

I learned later that not only had the surgeon tied my tubes (which was the "minor" surgery I had entered the hospital to have) but also found a cyst on an ovary. Out it came. And my uterus, while he was in the vicinity, looked like it needed to have a D & C. Which he did. And the uterine wall was punctured and I began hemorrhaging.

"We need your permission to remove your wife's uterus," the doctor explained to a befuddled husband, who was waiting to take me home after the "routine" procedure. "We've run into a problem, and we're giving her a transfusion right now."

And permission was given, and transfusion was given, and I was aware of something going on.

Call it an "out of body experience" or "near-death experience" if you will, but I saw and heard everything. I felt nothing. No pain, nothing. Rather than being alarmed, my reaction was something like: "Hmmm. This is very interesting. I wonder what's happening." I didn't "float" above my own body, but I was curiously detached. There were too many persons in the operating room for this to be a "routine" procedure, too, I concluded.

When I woke later that evening, a gentle recovery room nurse soothed my first attempts at conversation. "We're getting a room ready for you now."

I opened my dry, swollen lips and mumbled: "Room? I'm supposed to go home."

I think they knocked me out rather than argue with me, because the next time I was conscious, the doctor was leaning over me in my very own hospital room.

"We had a little problem," he began.

"I know," I said. "I saw and heard it all."

"You must have come out of the anesthesia briefly."

I shook my head. "No. I didn't hurt. I saw and heard everything."

Shaking his head, he mumbled a few phrases I'm sure he meant to assure me I had been dreaming, and exited the room.

I, on the other hand, knew absolutely, positively I was aware of what was going on. I didn't know it at the time, but this was to be the beginning of believing my own body, mind and spirit over that of a learned doctor.

A few weeks after the hysterectomy, I felt absolutely wonderful, invigorated, euphoric, and didn't need any sleep, thank you very much. I ate ravenously, yet lost weight. Finally, after noticing my hands shook all the time, I was convinced that maybe I should pay a visit to the family doctor.

"Are you taking speed?" he asked bluntly.

"Of course not," I huffed. ("My husband is the chemically dependent person in the family," I wanted to say.)

"Well, you're almost ready to stroke out. I'm sending you to a specialist. Right away."

The specialist determined I had hyperthyroidism and sent me to a radiologist, whereby after drinking a radium cocktail, my thyroid was dissolved. We took off to Aspen, Colorado, for a few weeks' vacation, where all I could manage to do was sleep; I didn't want to eat, *couldn't* eat, yet I returned home ten pounds heavier. Then it was time to begin thyroid replacement therapy.

This marriage limped along until 1982, and although I mourned the loss of another marriage, I was much too busy to grieve properly.

I didn't want or need the huge house, with its accompanying problems, so I moved to an apartment. I also went to the local community college and brushed up on my typing and business machines so I could get a job.

Never one to do things in half-measures, I threw myself into work and dating, burning the candle at both ends for at least two years. Working as a "temp," I soon felt confident enough to apply for a full-time position at a new oil and gas exploration company.

I also quickly had a steady boyfriend, too, and thought my life was finally back on track.

However, the oil company folded and my boyfriend rode off into the sunset with someone else. I promptly took another job and another boyfriend, thank you very much.

Another oil and gas company, a boyfriend pretty much like the first one...but I consoled myself by taking a trip with a couple of women friends to Hawaii.

And what does one do in Hawaii? Why, bask in the sun, of course. One of the worst things I could have done, so I found out later...but I didn't know then I was developing a disease that would warn against sunbathing.

Upon my return, you guessed it, this oil company also folded and this boyfriend also departed.

I began feeling some fatigue, so tired I could hardly get out of bed. I returned to the specialist who had treated my hyperthyroidism, and he suggested I might have a hormone imbalance—"Why don't you try taking Provera?" he suggested, writing out the prescription, which I dutifully had filled.

A bell should have gone off in my head, if not my doctor's. Since it is believed that lupus can be triggered by an excess of hormones, and this was the third hormone that my body was now being asked to process, I believe it was too much. It was totally unnecessary for me to have taken that drug. But at the time, I didn't question my doctor.

I do now.

Two months later, my symptoms began...

I woke up with my fingers so swollen I couldn't make my morning pot of coffee. I visited my family doctor, who pronounced, "Looks like arthritis." He prescribed an anti-inflammatory, which didn't work.

I then noticed a vague aching in arms, as if I had carried heavy books all day.

Then the swelling of hands. Wrists involved next; nieces playing with my watch and bracelet was excruciating. Extreme fatigue and weight loss. Rash on "V" neck, fiery red as though I had been in the sun a very long time.

My family practitioner was at a loss—"Probably just arthritis. After all, at your age…."

My relationship with a handsome businessman was ending. Charming, financially secure, we took many trips. But I was constantly on alert. Wondering where he was and who he was with. I called it off.

Still smarting from my divorce, this was a double blow. My muscles tensed constantly, and I sought relief in aspirin and another romance. Of course. I was burning the candle at both ends; I knew it, but I couldn't help myself.

The intensity of my physical pain increased to the point that nothing was alleviating it.

By now, I was working for a sole practitioner attorney, who specialized in workers' compensation and personal injury. I was struggling with the incredible fatigue, joint pain and swelling. Incredible pain, all over my body. My wrists were on fire, my knees swollen to the size of grapefruit. And nothing helped. Not aspirin, Advil, hot baths. Nothing.

On top of all this, we soon moved the office to a new location where we would be the first tenants and other offices would be built literally around us. The sole practitioner immediately took off for New Damn Mexico, as I began to call it under my breath, leaving me solely responsible for the whole moving process.

While workers were literally building around me all day long, I breathed fumes from paints, lacquers, varnish and carpet glue, not to mention cringing at the ear-splitting screams of sheet metal being cut and drills boring into concrete.

The attorney told me he thought I had carpal tunnel syndrome and would have to have surgery and then I wouldn't be able to type for a while. (And then he would have to let me go, I thought. He's all heart.)

I again went to my primary care physician who prescribed Feldene and told me to come back if I didn't get better.

I didn't.

I need to see somebody who knows what's going on, I thought. I asked a friend of a friend who was the wife of a physician. She ought to know.

"Dr. Charles Smith" (the true identity of all doctors in this narrative have been changed) she suggested. "He's expensive, but he's good."

I didn't care, at this point, now, with my knees being a prime target. I would see him at any price.

After an extensive examination, Dr. Smith intoned, "It is my considered opinion that you have lupus. I have no proof, so we will have to run some lab tests. In the meantime," he said, writing out the first of many prescriptions, "no more Naprocin. We'll use an anti-malarial drug that works well on lupus. It will take three months for it to begin working," he said, "but the pain will be lessened."

"Okay, great!"

"But there are some side effects," he cautioned.

"What side effects?"

"It affects the eyes. Your vision could be affected."

"You mean, as in blind? I could go blind?"

"I need for you to have a visual field base checkup, and then you must have your eyes examined every six months."

He turned his attention to a nurse who was chatting with another patient in the hallway outside the examining room, and proceeded to berate her for making too much noise.

As I paid my exorbitant bill, I pondered this new medication and its effects, filled the prescription at my friendly neighborhood pharmacy (the pharmacist and I would become very good friends through the years) and went back to the office, where our clerk was anxiously awaiting my diagnosis.

"Well," I began, "there's good news and there's bad news. The good news is, this new medicine should take effect in about three months and then the pain will be gone. The bad news is, this same medicine might cause me to go blind.

"Some choice," I wailed. "I can either hurt or go blind."

When I went home that evening, I reported by telephone to the friend who had sent me to Dr. Smith.

"He's strange. I don't know if he knows what he's doing, either. He said it is his 'considered opinion' that I have lupus. Well, either I do or I don't. I d like to know for sure and he can't tell me for sure. I'll give him three visits, and then I'm seeing somebody else," I said firmly.

And I meant it. This doctor was squirrelly as hell, and even as bad as I felt, I didn't want to waste any more time with him than I absolutely had to. No diagnosis, no relief from my pain, or I was out of there.

One night, I was overcome with pain, and my throat was "closing up." I couldn't breathe well. I called a friend, certain that lupus had swollen even my air passages, and I was about to die from lack of oxygen.

She rushed me to the emergency room, where I demanded a cortisone shot. I knew they worked, short term, from previous experiments by my various doctors. I made myself obnoxious by shouting, "I probably have lupus and I need a cortisone shot. *Now.*"

I congratulated myself on my assertiveness (actually I was downright hostile.) I was beginning to treat myself, as I had been told in the very beginning of seeking a diagnosis.

"If it is lupus, it will be a 'Do-I-Yourself' disease. *You* must chart your *own* recovery."

My friend took me home where I slept, pain-free, for the remainder of the night.

As I took the medication for the third month, and my pain had not been lessened, I was true to my word…I was Out of There.

Alternative Medicine:
I See a Reflexologist

I began asking other friends who they would recommend as a specialist—a diagnostician. And another friend sent me to see a reflexologist. She quickly became my friend. My guru, who literally "straightened me out." After seeing her, I walked easier, felt no pain.

"You don't have rheumatoid arthritis," she agreed.

I experimented with my reflexologist's diet, and found that when I avoided sugar, potatoes, tomatoes and red meat, my pain eased.

"Relax. Change your diet. And drink lots of water. What you have is environmental. An allergy to paint fumes, glues, and so forth. Stuff in the air…."

I went "Boing."

I told her about the new office. New carpet. Glue. Varnish. Faint fumes. Noise from downs the hail where new space was being built.

"Your immune system is fighting all that," she nodded. "You have to quit your job."

Of course, I couldn't quit my job. Even though the environment was hurting me; even though I hated it.

I was too scared.

I soon drained my savings account paying for these wonderful treatments and then I couldn't see her any more.

Other Various Therapies, Treatments: Visual Therapy

I attended a workshop on visual therapy—I was urged to let the child in me draw and paint, willy-nilly, then to draw how I would conquer my disease.

I drew an angel with a large golden sword, who touched me on various places of my body, sending a brilliant golden light searing through the cells, infusing them with holy light. I am kneeling in front of the angel, whom I named Andra, out of my subconscious, and there was no doubt about the name. Not Andrea, not Andrew, but Andra. My guardian angel.

Shortly after this course ended, I was strolling in the mall with my boyfriend du jour when I spotted a print I had had as a small child over my bed at my grandmother's house. I'm sure everyone is familiar with it: A guardian angel guides two small children across a wooden bridge, over a raging stream, while lightning flashes in the background.

When I mentioned this to an aunt at a family gathering, she snorted, "Well, I don't know why you think you were so crazy about that painting. When you were a little girl, you were always afraid the bridge would break."

Oh, me of little faith!

It currently hangs in my grandchildren's bedroom and I smile every time I see it.

I GO TO COUNSELING.

Somewhere, in some dusty archive bin, there is a videotape of me sobbing my heart out to a patient Brite Divinity School graduate. I agreed to the taping because (1) the price of counseling was just right (as I recall, almost free) (2) the location and times were convenient for me and (3) I really had no other choice at the time. We determined (1) that I had felt abandoned as a child, (2) fell into verbally and spiritually abusive relationships; (3) I have a really crappy disease that nobody understands and I'm angry about it. Finally, I was surprised to learn that I am stronger than I thought. All the women in my family history have been strong women. So why not me? I was assured I would survive this crisis. It was right on time, since my time for counseling was up.

READING SUCH BOOKS AS *LOVE, MEDICINE AND MIRACLES*.

I found I had to have faith that I would get better. Incident after incident was displayed in front of me. If they can do it, why can't I?

BIOFEEDBACK AT THE EASTER SEALS.

I almost blew out the equipment the poor counselor put on my arm. Well, it's their own fault....I was told to think about my ex-husband. Bells and whistles went off the charts. Intrigued, the counselor tried it again, and again the equipment registered extreme stress reactions. Not that I had to have a machine tell me this, but this was proof that my thinking/emotions/subconscious was literally making me sick. I was then instructed to think about something tranquil and soothing, and to breathe slowly and deeply. Almost no movement on the chart. So I *can* control my body's reaction to stressful thoughts.

Doctor #2
I See a Female Physician

"Go see Evelyn Brown," a friend suggested, when I told her my story. "She's a rheumatologist." I thought, *She might understand the pain I'm in, and being a woman, she wouldn't brush it off as psychosomatic.*

I hobbled into her office one raw, rainy morning, knees swollen to the point where it was difficult to walk. I had been getting up at 5 a.m. to soak in a tub of hot water, eat breakfast so I could take the pills that weren't doing me any good, so I could get to work by 8 a.m.

Today was especially troublesome.

"Hop right up here, Ms. Morris." Her nurse patted the examination table, high as Mt. Everest to me at that point.

"*Hop?*" I said. "You're asking me to *hop up?*"

She flushed, and then softened. "Here's a step stool; it should be a little easier for you."

She left the room and returned a moment later with the interminable paperwork. "Dr. Brown will be in to see you in a few minutes."

I diligently filled in all the blanks while seated on the high examining table, legs dangling (surely this can't do my knees a whole lot of good, I speculated) and wondering why it was that I had to put on this flimsy paper gown when all that needed to be looked at was my knees. Today, that is, although I still hurt in every joint in my body, today it was the knees that suffered the most.

As I finished the last question on the lengthy paperwork, the door opened and the renowned Dr. Evelyn Brown entered.

She went straight to the point.

Her point.

"What beautiful swollen knees!" she rhapsodized, poking at them none too gently.

"Do they hurt?"

Do they hurt? I barely restrained myself from yelling out loud. Of course they hurt! I must have said something to that effect, or else she read my leap toward the ceiling as proof enough that yes, I was hurting.

"Hot," she said briskly. "Your joints are hot. Especially first thing in the morning. I'll prescribe hot paraffin for you…you could soak your hands in it on wakening."

And I was treated to a hot paraffin treatment that very day. I dipped my hands into hot, melted wax, withdrawing them to cool and harden. Moments later, the nurse removed the wax, and my hands indeed felt better and were less stiff.

"This works for rheumatoid arthritis," Dr. Brown chirped. "You probably have rheumatoid arthritis."

What? Didn't she know either? I wondered. Another round of medications. Another round of waiting to see whether they would work or not.

As I departed her office that morning, it dawned on me that I needed treatment more for my *knees* than for my *hands*, for goodness sakes. And my poor "beautiful, swollen knees" were still the same.

I gave this latest medical treatment a couple of months, with no success, and no resolution for the pain in my *knees*, she at last threw up her hands and said the words "Gold Treatment."

I couldn't afford to take off work every week for several hours for office visits, I told her. My job was hanging on the ragged edge, as my focus on my physical pain had caused me to make several minor errors on office paperwork, and The Sole Practitioner had given me warning.

I was once again Out of There.

A Few Words About Depression and Treatment, or
The MHMR Marching Band

What I didn't know at the time was, I was in a depression, brought on by the disease itself (anyone who deals with a chronic illness has a "built-in depression factor") and I was, indeed, "let go."

Once again, I'm out of work.

What am I going to do?

Why, find something else, of course.

In the meantime, I began a search to treat the depression that was descending on me like a shroud. My cognitive functions had deteriorated to the point that when I read something, I couldn't remember what I had just read. Not a good thing in a working environment.

Since I was unemployed, and virtually broke, I had to go to Mental Health and Mental Retardation Agency: MHMR. This would be the beginning of the Alphabet Jungle, consisting of acronyms such as TRC, WC, TWCC, TRC, TCJC, HEB, and many other agency abbreviations.

I had a terrible time finding the damn place: First of all, the Summit Clinic is not on Summit Avenue. Oh, it used to be, but they just kept the name when they moved, the clerk at the desk chirped.

The MHMR was located, predictably, in the poorest, worst, "bad" part of town.

I parked my car in a junk-filled lot near vacant buildings with broken windows; it looked like a war zone.

I entered the deteriorating building cautiously, inspecting the peeling gray paint on the walls, half-expecting a rodent to run across my foot.

Upstairs, I decided; the businesses and agencies on this floor were not related to MHMR.

Should I climb the stairs or enter the elevator?

If I take the stairs, my knees will be screaming. But I don't want to get into the elevator and be assaulted in private.

I opt for the elevator, anyway. It creaks and groans its way to the second floor. I remain alone in the elevator, thank God.

I emerge to see a sign on 2nd floor that says MHMR.

But a cheerful clerk tells me I'm in the wrong place.

"Go up one more floor."

Grumbling to myself, and wondering what the hell I was doing here in the first place, I trudged up the flight of stairs.

I entered a gray waiting room where stale body odors assaulted me and sat gingerly in the on one of the gray-blue plastic chairs placed on soiled gray carpet.

It's miserably hot in here.

I read the signs all over the walls: "Do Not Park in the grocery store lot. Your car will be towed."

"Bring all meds with you to next appt."

Gray People shuffle in.

The Retarded. The Hostile.

Some tell silent jokes to themselves. Irritable mothers, hyper grown children.

The staff here deserves a medal.

Finally, it's my turn to see the doctor.

He is weary-looking.

He asks questions, ending with:

"Ever felt like killing someone?"

"Not yet."

He scribbles on a pad.

I get a diagnosis.

"Adjustment disorder."

And a prescription for Pamelor.

As I am leaving, a nurse comes up to young man who is rocking back and forth, telling incomprehensible jokes to himself.

She hands his silent, drawn mother a bottle of pills.

"These will help his delusional states. Have him take two at lunch and two at dinner."

She says this right in the open. In front of everybody. Of

course, here, there can be no secrets.

Everybody here is crazy.

Except me.

Another Day, Another Job....
And
Doctor #3

So I next went to work as a secretary in the management office of a large urban mall.

I lasted at that job about as long as I had lasted with Dr. Smith.

And I was still hurting.

I would try another job, and someone else, thank you.

That Someone would be at St. Joseph's Hospital

Dr. Green more or less shrugged after extensive tests: "I don't find anything definitive." (A "diagnosis" I was destined to hear over and over again.)

So I would be directed to University of Texas Southwest Medical Center. Surely at this prestigious teaching hospital, a diagnosis would be found.

Somewhere along here, it gets a little strange. (As if it weren't strange enough!) I kept thinking about a woman I had known several years earlier. At odd moments, while I'm driving, not thinking about much of anything.

She had lupus.

She had died of lupus.

Why was I thinking about her? We were not close. We worked together at the museum (as volunteers). In fact, I thought she was rather "crabby"—now I was beginning to see why.

Pain makes you crabby.

Why did I suddenly think of her? Could it be that I really did have lupus, but nobody knows it but me? Does this mean I'm going to die?

"Not today," I muttered grimly, as I swung my car into the

parking lot at UT Southwestern in Dallas.

"We tested you for SLE," the doctor told me. She was the finest rheumatologist around. Yet she said, "We found nothing conclusive."

How many times had I heard those or similar words "We can't find anything definitive."

I returned to the law office where I had begun working after leaving the shopping mall job, diagnosis of "Connective Tissue Disorder" in hand.

Since I had spent more time out of the office than they felt was reasonable, I was summarily dismissed.

The journal entries begin. (Feel free, by the way, to skip over parts you aren't interested in, or feel like you've read before. Some entries are mundane, talk of work and school and family, but I needed to remind myself that life goes on around me, ordinary tasks of the day need to be taken care of and my entries also reflect my friends' care and concern, with outings to movies, dinners, etc. So if sometimes I repeat myself, blame lupus lapse.)

I decided to keep a journal reflecting my daily bouts with the disease of lupus. If you think there are an enormous amount of entries, you should have seen those that I cut! Many seem repetitive, but that's what I was feeling at that time in this battle with lupus. I chose to personify this disease with the name of "Lupe"—and she takes on the persona of a gypsy, moving at whim throughout my body, setting up camp some days in my knees, other days in my wrists...and always, she builds campfires, stoking them, tending them carefully, unmindful of the pain these fires are causing me.

Lupe is actually a quite remarkable woman. She is vivacious, fiery (pardon the pun), flashy, an independent, gutsy sort of girl. Lupe has steadfastly refused to tell me why she has chosen my body to explore, nor will she listen to my pleas to vacate the premises. She just hums softly to herself, stirs the ashes of her campfire, and sits back to gaze into the smoke.

This past week, old Lupe was in her finest hours. She traveled quickly, all over my body, building campfires and then moving on to a new spot. The weather was cold, sleet hitting the windowpanes, and the wind howled to get in.

Lupe was not, by God, going to get cold. She moved rapidly and her fires kept her warm.

I protested when my knees swelled so badly I couldn't walk or get up from the couch. I became most angry with Lupe; however, the night I attempted to take a hot tub bath, and ended up climbing into the tub, trying to turn around and sit down, and ended up facing "the wrong way."

Well, I thought that was funny, and I began to laugh. Lupe, however, was insulted, and made me cry. I told her how much I hated her presence in my life and all she did was shrug, and remind me that I still had to climb out of the tub, so I'd better save my strength.

3/18/88 Saturday p.m.

There is a struggle going on inside myself. I don't know what it's all about, but I know it hurts.

I have been no stranger to pain these last two years. I wake every morning with the same disease I went to bed with the night before...no miracles occurred during my restless sleep.

The physical pain will be there, I'm told, forever, unless or until I have a remission. And I can cope with the physical pain, I believe. Better than the accompanying depression that seems to cry out at night and to greet me first thing each morning.

I hurt. I don't want to move and make it hurt any more. *Depression tells me to stay still. Don't get up and go to work. Don't do your meditations, your reading, take the phone calls from your friends. Depression tells me I'm always going to feel used-up, burned out, crippled.*

3/21/88 Monday p.m.

I cried a bit, finally. Shit happens. But that doesn't mean I don't get to hurt. I just have to stand there. I can't run. I have to walk through it.

3/31/88

What a bitch of a few days. Tuesday morning Mr. H called me into his office and told me, more or less, that "the workload was heavy" and he knew I had days "when you're not feeling well" so he said, "I thought you and Anna could trade places." I agree. Who can handle that desk, anyway?

But deep down, I feel like I had not done a good job. Hell, nobody can do that desk—they've tried. So why do I think I can?

Anyway, I feel embarrassed. Even had a dream that I was naked from the waist down. Bare-assed. I feel shame. None of that is reality. The reality is, my workload is now easier even though I feel incompetent trying to learn another new job. Does that make me stupid? No. Only human.

I felt abandoned, one more time. So Mr. H abandoned me. Two husbands, boyfriends abandoned me. Is that true? Did I cause it? No, of course not.

But it's time to see a counselor again. I don't know how I can afford it.

It's difficult to go to work and hold my head up after everyone knows I've been "demoted."

Ostensibly, they have offered me a less stressful situation— and it is. I still have the same salary, plus when we start on the 18th, an increase of $125 a month.

But I'm tired of hurting. I want an end to my pain. Both kinds. I want to—what? Grow up? Learn to live?

I know I have to take care of myself. But I don't know how. I thought I did, but if I did, why am I feeling so bereft now? Why can't I feel good about myself and my work?

My rebellious child is kicking me.

4/8/88

Fear has set in. I was "talked to" at work. About the quality of my work. I worry. I can't seem to do anything right. All negative thoughts flood my mind: I'm a failure.

And, yes, I'm let go...Again.

Diagnosis at Last!

October 1988

Job-wise, I kept taking the same action, expecting different results.

Went to temporary work (Hampton) more of the same. Was put on the health plan, which led me to the doctor who diagnosed my baffling illness. Dr. Dan. He asked me if I were part Indian.

"Yes, I am. My grandmother was half Indian."

He nodded. "North American Indians (or Native Americans) are particularly susceptible to lupus. I used to work at the Indian Hospital in Oklahoma, and I saw a lot of it. We'll get some blood work done…"

I sighed. Would there be anything to see? Another time of waiting, wondering and hurting.

The blood work came back.

And the little monster had shown up.

"It's lupus."

"Thank God," I breathed. "Now we know what it is. Now we can treat it."

He told me my reaction was typical. After all this time…an answer.

I was prescribed cytoxan and prednisone.

Where There's a Will There's a Burial Plot

I tell my family I have lupus—what it can do to me. They are puzzled, they are afraid. They are angry. They are helpless.

Except for my kids…they buy a burial policy for me. Not exactly what I would want as a gift, but I am touched.

And I begin writing my will. Such as it is.

Mostly, I sigh, my children will inherit my debts.

However, it was almost a case of "too little, too late."

By February of the next year, I was in the hospital.

November 1988

He can't do this to me, can he? What led me to the hospital…

I received a letter from my ex-husband, Doug. "I will no longer be sending you the monthly check, as we owe the IRS and I am taking that sum out of our community funds."

That was all.

I am stunned. Heartsick. I want to throw up. I am scared. I am angry, furious. I call my sponsor. I cry. Nothing I can do about it—except—sue him.

Letter to an Ex-husband

Do you think you can hurt me, still?
After you left me and took up with Her
And danced away without another thought
Of the chaos you left behind?
No, my former partner, you cannot hurt me
Any more. I won't give you the power to do so.
I used to give you power, you know.
That you didn't deserve and that you misused,
And I've learned never to do that again.
When I think of how I trusted you
And you betrayed that trust,
I wonder how you an live with yourself
And how can anyone live with you?
What goes around, comes around
Are you ready for the inevitable?
While I, my former partner, gladly
Greet each new experience with a clean conscience
And don't have to look over my shoulder
To see who's watching me.
To God, re: my ex-husband:
God, I want to be free from revenge.
I don't want my heart to be hardened.
I want to be able to forgive the poor sick man
For being exactly what he is, a poor, sick man.
Part of me wants to scream, shout at him
And call him names.
Part of me wants to carry around this anger and hurt and
        indignation
Like some kind of damn battle flag: "Look what he did
        to me."

41

Nobody cares what he did to me.
Least of all him.
Part of me says, let it go and forget it.
And which part I feel
Depends on my closeness to You

1/4/89

Winter of My Discontent

Winter.
Cat sleeps
Curled against the cold.
Wind chimes clank
And clang and bang
At each blast of icy air.
No music here.
Just discord.
I contemplate the leaden sky
And turn on the electric blanket
And fix soup for supper
And cat sleeps,
Oblivious to my preparations.
Why can't I be more like my cat?
Rest assured that all will be well.
Cold may come
And dark skies threaten
And cat sleeps on.
Depression is part of lupus,
I understand.
Whether it's the medication
Or just a mood swing,
It doesn't matter.
I hate being depressed.
Even just a little bit.
For a little while.
It's really not "that bad"—
It falls on me
Like a dead weight

And I must heed its call.
I am immobilized,
Watching TV.
And not really watching
What I'm watching.
That's the worst it gets,
And that's not bad.
I could do worse, I suppose.
I know it won't last.
I call a few friends
And discover others
Worse off than me.
It doesn't help much.
Depression has its own hold on me.
I know it's okay,
It will pass…
But being depressed
Depresses me.

Undated

I hate this disease. I feel like I don't deserve the pain and inconvenience it causes. I don't like being different from other people. I feel like a child who can't run and play with the other kids. I feel financially burdened, barely able to keep going, everybody wanting a piece of me and not enough of me to go around.

I feel like I want to be "rescued" from my creditors. I think sometimes that if I had enough money to pay my bills, I would feel better, that even this lupus would go away.

I don't know what to tell my parents about how I feel. I don't want to burden them with worry, but I need their help, too. I don't want to be a child who begs for nickels and dimes to go to the movies.

I wish God would give me a full-time job and the strength to do it. In a way, He has. And I know that. My feeling is that it's just not enough.

Thank you very much, God, but it isn't. I have to keep asking and it seems like it's never enough. Yet I know it really is...please help me to see this.

I'm scared, God. I think about dying a lot. Well, not a lot, but at odd times. I don't want to die because of this disease, thank you. If I had my way—I'd be an old lady in good health, who just passes away in her sleep.

But I won't get to choose my manner of death. I can, however, choose my manner of living. I choose to live each day the best way I can. I treasure my friends, my family, and wish there were more time for them. I miss my children and wish I could be with them more. I have to remember that they have their own lives and not to burden them unnecessarily with my disease.

I want this lupus to just go away and leave me alone. I want the doctors and medical bills and the blood tests to just fade away into oblivion. I want to bargain with God—think if I'm a good girl, He'll make me "all better." I also know God expects me to take care of this stuff as best as I can.

Okay, so I'll pay my bills, as best as I can. I'll go in for the blood tests, and keep working at whatever God puts in my way, and keep loving my friends and family and continue to be honest with them.

January 1989

A Job with a National Oil & Gas Company Playing Lease Rentals Secretary

I had found another "permanent" job in the oil and gas industry. With benefits, taking preexisting conditions. I double-checked before accepting the job.

Due to a change in my HMO coverage with this company, I was obliged to find another doctor who was under the Sanus program: Dr. Larry Morton was recommended by 'Dr. Dan.'

3/14/89

New Rheumatologist I see Larry Morton
W/126; diff. w/knees; TMJ; V rash on neck....
Prednisone 5 mg. Plaquenil 200 mg; off Orudis 2 weeks

Well, Lupe! Seems like I got the best of you, after all. Am cleaning house, bit by bit. Trying not to overdo. Even on guard against her sneak attacks. Made a vow that I won't go through another day like Sat. when I felt and acted so crippled. Everyone notices and I hate it.

Everyone wanted to know about lupus. What can I say? It's like RA? Joints hurt, a lot. Constantly. Sometimes worse than others. It's a bitch. Do I sound whiney? Do I sound angry? Do I sound like a damn martyr? I have to find some better answers.

Sunday a.m.

Feel like I need to sweat. I feel better when I can let out all those toxins. The smoke from Lupe's campfires.

Ah, sleep on, ol' Lupe. Even you can't last forever. You have to have your rest and sleep and you are no match for medication, rest and determination to get rid of you.

You may win some battles, but I will win the war.

3/20/89

Went to my regular monthly checkup with my new rheumatologist (new job, new health insurance = new doctor.) I told him I had a funny pain in my shoulder blade, on the left side. Temp. 103 in office.

He took a chest x-ray and told me, "Go home and pack a bag. Better yet, get someone to do it for you."

"Why?"

"Because you're going to the hospital."

45

"No I'm not." (Denial is a wonderful thing.)

"Yes, you are. You have pneumonia."

I was dumbfounded. I hadn't coughed. I had no problem breathing.

I just had a funny little pain...

I called my brother's wife and told her I was checking into the hospital and to please pick up a few things at my house.

I then drove myself to the hospital—typical of me.

I stood stoically at the registration desk, my knees shaking, until someone shoved a wheelchair under me.

By the time I got upstairs and into my bed, I was almost convulsing. IVs were started (massive doses of antibiotics and cortisone) and I finally realized I was *one sick puppy*.

I was in the hospital four or five days.

Friends got word and came by. Mercifully, they did not comment on my dreadful appearance, or the tubes inserted in various parts of my body.

My head sweat profusely; my pillowcase was continually wet. Nurses came and went, gave me meds, changed my pillowcases, sheets, and let me sleep, which was all I wanted. Meals were unappetizing, I had little appetite, and I was shaky when I stood up to go to the bathroom.

A shower felt wonderful. I stood under the hot spray as long as I could, until a watchful nurse knocked on the door and asked me to come out. That was okay with me; my knees were giving out under me.

Blurred days and nights. IVs were changed. Pills and more pills. Blood drawn. Go ahead, I thought. Take what you want. I don't care. I really don't.

Someone called the chaplain.

Was I that obvious?

It was a woman. Good.

She asked me to tell her what I was feeling.

"Besides pain?" I mumbled.

"Yes. Besides physical pain."

"I don't want to have this disease," I began, and to my utter horror, tears welled in my eyes and cascaded down my feverish cheeks.

"Tell me about it," she urged.

And I did.

"Well," she said when I finally paused, "it's a bad disease. But you know you're going to be all right, don't you?"

"For now," I shot back. I instantly regretted my cynicism. "Yes, I will."

And this time, I believed it.

"Thank you for coming," I said.

She smiled and left the room as I fell into a deep, restful sleep.

My parents arrived and "flapped" for a couple of days, coming and going. When I was released, and was back in my own home, they alternated between "hovering," anxiously watching my every move, or they did nothing at all.

4/17/89 Monday

I returned to work. I needed my job.

But Lord, I was weak and tired. And I had somehow developed a limp, of all things. My right leg was dragging behind me. Still, I trudged on.

Entering my supervisor's office one morning, I stepped out of my shoe and fell flat on my face.

Not a cool thing to do.

I lost that job, too. Lupus was mentioned at my "exit interview" shortly afterward, and I thought about suing them, but was too exhausted to begin a lawsuit.

Now both my legs weren't working right. My ankles weren't bending.

I had vasculitis.

As I left the building, for the last time, escorted out, no less, like a common thief (*so I won't sabotage any equipment, or take anything with me, I knew, nothing personal*) hurricane winds blew across the park. The trees bent horizontally, to the ground. I stood against the wind, wondering if I would literally be knocked down. I struggled forward to my car. The wind ceased as suddenly as it had started.

God sent that wind for me....

To let me know I can weather the storm?

I was numb all the way home. How I got there, I'll never know.

There was no God. Or, if there was, He had abandoned me.

One more time, I had no job.

I felt less than.

I wanted to die.

But my friends wouldn't let me.

So I cried, yelled, beat my bed with a plastic baseball bat, as I had been encouraged to do in therapy, and hated everybody in the world, and myself, most of all, which had not been encouraged in therapy.

Despair settles in like a fog over me. Grief for who I thought I was wrapped me in a shroud. Most of all, fear gripped me in its iron jaws.

I can't survive this blow. I can't do anything. I'm going to lose my house, everything I own. My pride is nonexistent.

Monday night comes and goes I'm still alive. I eat dinner. I move. I breathe. I talk to others who support me...who sustain me, who live for me. Who believe in me.

I tell my parents I may have to live with them. They tell me I can, they have offered before.

My kids call. They love me. They offer money, a place to live.

I am exhausted enough to sleep.

4/18/89

Dr. appt. Need a brace for my foot

Wt. 116

Feet drop r foot.

Pred. 50 mg. Put on Buspar PRN

Dr. says they shouldn't have fired me. Too bad, but they did, I think.

Tuesday is a blur. I am in shock, I guess.

Wednesday. I have an interview at City Hall. I sparkle. I tell

48

them what they want to hear. The man I interview with looks angry. I make a mental note of that.

Job sounds interesting, with all kinds of "big wigs" but stressful. I make a mental note of that. I don't need any more stress.

I leave City Hall. Go check on Unemployment. Any left at TEC? All gone. Well. Too early to file on the National Oil Company. Besides, it's not worth the hassle.

I need to go back to Hampton Hospital Corp. and rejoin the temporary pool.

So I go and eat lunch at the Plaza Café. Soothing. Take my physical.

Stop by doctor's office to check on where to get my leg brace. Dr. and I meet in hallway. He tells me not to worry. He has spoken to Lauri, who called earlier, and calmed her fears.

Went to atty's office and got a copy of the letter to Doug.

Oh, yeah—I'm suing him for non-payment of contractual alimony. Leave my attorney a note re my job, the brace, disability ins., etc.

I get home, get the mail. A birthday card from parents: "You're still our little girl," and a $25 check. Wishing they could do more.

A card from dear friend and $30 cash.

Well, it's too much. I cry like a baby.

Exhausted, I take the phone off the hook; lie down on the couch and nap.

A half-hour later, Evelyn and Katie appear at my door. She brings in four sacks of groceries: eggs, coffee, bread, prepared food; rice, toilet paper...and puts it all away for me.

I am overcome.

Mom and Dad call.

Terri sends money.

There is a God.

Thursday

I put up my winter clothes. Do laundry. Meet Joyce for dinner. I am reasonably sane. I am safe. I have a check for the bank. I have the promise of work. I have put an ad in the paper for a roommate. I have some time to make some decisions.

It wouldn't be bad to move.

I can keep working at Hampton and other temps to take enough to live. I'll just have to cut expenses...meaning, lower rent. Apartments aren't bad, if I get the right one for me.

I don't need this house. I need a place to live. Period. I don't need a "powerful" job. I need a job to provide for my needs. Period.

4/20/89 3 a.m.

Down Again

God, why do I have lupus? This was not part of my plan for me.

I feel punished, somehow, for some unknown transgression. What did I do wrong? Or what did I leave undone?

Was it in my childhood that I displeased you or someone else? Did I harm someone by my anger? Was I really angry with you? They tell me we choose our own diseases, according to our needs. I must need to punish myself, somehow, by having my body turn against itself.

What kind of struggle is going on inside me that causes both physical and emotional pain? Is it the struggle to express myself?

Is it all those feelings inside that are causing me such pain? I'm learning to express myself and be honest and sharing with others.

Things are a little better with Mom and Dad today because I am risking telling them my feelings...*their* response is *their* problem.

If they let their fear get in the way of their feelings, they will act the same old way...brush it off, don't look at the problem, ignore it and it will go away. Don't ask questions.

50

But isn't that blaming your parents?

Let's play, "It's all their fault."

Wrong. *I* could have done different. If I hadn't been afraid.

Now I'm not afraid.

Now I'm talking, risking the same response, but getting different ones more often—hooray. Is this the beginning of a healing of some kind?

4/23/89

My doctor advised me that I might need a leg brace, but in order to help the vasculitis in my ankles right away I should sleep in high-topped tennis shoes. I went to Wal-Mart and in the boys' department found some red and white high-topped tennis shoes.

The first night I put them on to sleep in, I was in misery.

It was summer. They were hot. I ended up kicking them off during the night.

This would never do. A friend suggested that I make a game out of it. Air-condition those dudes.

I ruined my manicure scissors cutting "vents" into the sides of the sneakers; then I cut hearts and stars all over, and on one shoe with magic marker printed "Wonder Woman" and on the other shoe "Shazaam."

One night, while getting ready for bed, I happened to see myself in the full-length mirror on the back of the door. It reflects this outrageous creature without my wig, thin, wispy black hair sticking out in odd directions from a nearly bald head; moon face devoid of contouring makeup; unmascara-ed eyes wide with fear; pale arms and legs incongruously thin against a thickening body bloated from prednisone—a body that was clad in a white cotton gown with lace on the waltz length hem; and, beneath the flounce, *those red, high-top boys' tennis shoes.*

I gazed at this pathetic creature and it gazed back, and suddenly, I began to laugh.

And so did the reflection. We laughed until we were breathless, this crazed-looking woman, and then we trundled off

51

to bed, wrestling the red, high-topped tennis shoes into position against the makeshift footboard, and falling into a deep sleep.

Somehow, I knew this was a sign of mental, if not physical, health.

I return home from visiting my friend Virgie at All Saints Hospital, where she is ill. I feel warm. Almost feverish. My arm has a rash as if pinpricks/broken blood vessels. Have Dr. apt. tomorrow a.m. anyway.

I'm taking an art class—part of my healing.

I drew my pictures as instructed—me and my disease. The Sword of Truth cutting out the bad cells and God's light flowing through me. Red blouse for anger working with me in the fight.

I had fun coloring like a kid.

4/24/89

Wt. 120
R foot drop
Continue Pred.60mg dec. To 30mg.
Put on Darvocet N-100 PRN

Up before the alarm goes off. Sense of well-being despite the shaking that begins the instant I stand up.

But thank God I can stand up. Today.

God, I have so many plans. I really want to live before I have to die. Don't take me too soon, please. But I know if it pleases you to take me home to you today, that would mean I've accomplished what you put me here to do. I'm still trying to discover what that is.

I believe part of my being alive and on this earth is to tell others of your love, evidenced by what has taken place in my life. How you have carried me through despair and destruction and kept me from evil. How you have taught me to love myself and others. How to accept love freely and give it back with no reservations.

I wonder if there is yet more purpose for me. Do I need to accomplish a great task?

I want to write again. I will do that. I intend to write my story for my children, anyway. My Army Brat days.

I Get "Stroke Shoes"

Between 10:30 and noon, I went to a specialty shoe store and bought two pair of shoes: sandals and a pair of bone colored lace-ups like my black ones.

I remember a friend of mine telling me about her experience with those type of shoes. She said a kid told her, "My aunt wore these after she had her stroke."

Thus, they became my "stroke shoes." Also a new pair of Keds, shoes to wear casually. Spent too much money.

Discontinued the Cytoxan in favor of Imuran. Don't like the side effects of Cytoxan.

Let's Play "Primary Care Physician Ping-Pong"

Believe I'll go back to Anderson and Marsh.

I stop at Ridgmar Square Apartments. Rent is too much.

My urine test at Hampton showed Darvocet and they said I didn't list it. I had to go show them the prescription bottle.

Tomorrow I will call re: handicapped sticker. Go to Social Security to see about disability.

4/25/89 Tuesday 6 a.m.

Woke easily and early. Slept well. Feeling of accomplishment helps. I ironed last night. Why do I feel like I have to accomplish something every day? Some task, a large task. Heck, it's enough of a task just to get up each day.

But I push.

I wish my leg wasn't in trouble. The imbalance makes me feel like I'm sick. Even when I walk through the house I feel—*invalided*. I worry about walking around in the "real" world.

I worry about my memory. Am I losing it? My eyes seem uncooperative at times, too. I felt warm yesterday. Took my temp at 9 p.m.—it was abut 99.5.

I hate the little blood vessels bursting in my left arm. Will this happen on my face?

How vain!

4/26/89

Woke thinking *I'm not a person with a disease. I am a whole person who happens to be diseased.* That is, not entirely well.

That makes a difference.

I'll check out more apts. today. Go to City Hall and apply for a word processing job. Sounds less stressful. But must remember: Ceaseless activity doesn't work.

4/27/89 5:30 a.m.

I found a lupus support group.

They asked us last night what makes us fatigued. Heck, I don't know! I don't even know when I'm tired until I drop over. I have to learn the early signs and stop before I get there. I'll have to ask someone to tell me. I think my inner dialogue in the past has been:

"I'm tired."

"No, you're not tired. You're just lazy. Now finish that monumental job within the next ten minutes. And when you're through with that, do the dishes. What a mess this place is...."

"I must be lazy, then."

Now I know...I'm not lazy. I am *tired.* Lupus makes me tired to begin with.

Worry makes me tired. (Money, moving, etc.)

Dishonest people make me tired...those who "blab" about nothing at all make me tired.

Procrastination makes me tired. The actual doing of the chore

54

makes me feel better, actually.

Pain is the biggest fatigue producer. If I can stay out of the pain—fighting the pain is so very hard. I have to remember to take some meds for the pain.

4/28/89

I am zonked. Woke at 5 a.m. and went back to sleep. First time I've done that since I started the mega doses of prednisone. Took a darvocet last night.

I keep getting into the future. I'm already moved into an apt. I thought this morning of what I said when I moved in here, Sept. 1983:

"I'm not moving again. They'll have to carry me out of here in the box." Little did I know this would almost become a self-filling prophecy.

It won't be so bad; I've got lots of help. But today is just today. I have enough to handle today.

Stress. It all boils down to how do I handle the stress of daily living. Not well, so far, is the answer.

Feel "fragmented" this morning. Emotionally hung over. Overloaded. Brain drain.

Well, some days are better than others.

4/28/89 p.m.

Had a sinking spell this evening. I did too much again.

Also need to take my pred on time and I was late…so my body went into a spin *and I started to cry.*

Damn this disease. I don't want to go through what I'm going through. It's too much. The financial worries—how am I going to support myself?

I'm tired of being brave. Tired of being tired. Tired of trying to explain this disease. (Maybe I just don't need to do that.)

I called one of the women at the lupus support group and asked her about the pred and my sudden mood changes. She said

I was correct. It's bad enough having lupus, taking all this medication and then have all these shitty circumstances dumped on top. No wonder I cratered.

Went to lunch with Liz. We wore ourselves out looking at apts.

I want to move/I don't want to move.

I want to be brave/I don't want to be brave.

I want to work Monday/I don't want to work on Monday…or Tuesday. Too many things going on.

I'm very warm. Have a bit of a fever. Ribs hurt. Must remember to take a darvocet before bed.

4/29/89 10:30 a.m.

Bob called for me to babysit Katie.

Mom and Dad called while I was there. They are concerned I wasn't working yet. I told them I was probably supposed to rest now. As I'd be working soon.

I hear their fear, too.

I wish all this was over. Sold the house, moved to the apt. and have a good steady job.

I have to grieve over my lost health. Part of me is gone. I'll never be the same again. Damn.

I've never liked change. I don't want to move. I want things to be the way they are. But the reality is, the way things are is awful. God wants me to move on. He's just not telling me where or when right now. I have to trust and follow Him.

Trust and obey.

But that is *so very hard* to do.

4/30/89 5 a.m.

Dreamed I was saying goodbye to another woman who looked in radiant health but who is ill. But I knew she was going to be okay. She "just needs to take it easy for a while."

How long is a while?

I got up and looked in the bathroom mirror and was startled to think: "*Look at that good-looking woman*" instead of "*Oh, God, I look awful; my cheeks are fat, my hair's a mess…*"

I looked as though I had all my makeup on and my hair looked good.…I even considered not washing it today but leaving it just the way it is.

I'm really concerned today about this foot problem. It slows me down (maybe it's supposed to?). I worry about moving and the problem I have just walking around.

How will I manage?

Stay out of the future.

4/30/89 5:49 a.m.

I have been "inflamed" by my responses to life. Inflammatory response in body = lupus.

Anger raged in me.

I can't have things my way.

Angry at myself.…I was never good enough. Why can't I/… Why didn't I.…You never…Shame on you…you dummy… You're not smart enough… you're not pretty enough. You can't keep a husband. You're not a good mother. You're a bad person. Don't show your anger; you may be abandoned. Be nice to everybody.

Try harder.…

What a bunch of lies I've been taught.

I sometimes fail and that's okay. I am a human *being*, not a human *doing*. I'm not dumb. I am a capable, resourceful and strong person. I am a survivor. I am not a victim of anything. Not even circumstances. I refuse to be a martyr.

I am a good mother. I love my children, as they are God's children. He gave them to me for a while and I have given them back into this hands.

I am not a bad person. I am a human, with human faults. I can now freely feel and show all my emotions, from grief to joy and not feel ashamed of them.

I don't have to be nice to everybody at my expense.

Instead of try harder, let go and let God.

4/30/89 10:30 p.m.

Tired, yet not ready for sleep. Virgie comes by. We went to eat Italian food. Came home tired.

The vasculitis has now invaded my left ankle. I have bruises on my arm; tingling.

I also noticed I have slight sunburn on my neck and shoulders. *A flare is going on.*

I hear "you look wonderful" all the time. To be so sick with such a disease as lupus—it's hard for people to believe I'm sick.

Closing doors is painful. I'm closing the door on this house. On my old self. And it's a grief process, one more time.

I *know* how to move, having done it all my life.

I *don't* know how to grieve over losses.

5/1/89

Wt. 119
Pred. 30 mg. Put on Cytoxan for vasculitis 50 mg.

5/1/89 7:30

After breakfast I immediately started shaking. Took pred. Hate this wired/tired feeling.

Just need to do the next right thing today. If that means take care of yourself, okay, then I can do that.

I'll have some guilt, though.

Old tapes: *You should be working. Why aren't you doing something? Are you trying to find another job? (How stupid a question is that?) Did you try...(*fill in the company name)?

5/1/89 5:16 p.m.

Lauri called. Wanted to know how I was doing. I told her about my left foot now. About going to see Dr. Morton and starting on Cytoxan. About how I'm not working yet. She mentioned—humorously—how Doug had kept her on a strict budget at school.

I told her I didn't want to talk about it.

I started to cry.

I told her I was tired and couldn't cope with talking about her father right now...and that if he hadn't done what he has done, I wouldn't be in such a bad financial shape right now.

She had to answer another phone, so we said goodbye. It was really awkward.

I want to be busy and do things, yet I'm so exhausted just walking around the house. I worry about falling. I have done everything I can to get work out of Hampton...it just isn't there.

I have also called two more temp agencies.

I picked up the papers for a handicapped sticker.

Tomorrow I'll pick up the papers for SS disability and SSI, when I file at TEC.

God, I'm so afraid. Afraid I can't work. Afraid I won't have insurance...afraid, period.

I read today that "Delay doesn't mean denial." I wish I could believe that.

I need to call my lawyer.

I need to call my congressman.

I need to let go and let God. One more time.

AMEX got real ugly this afternoon. Threatening to "serve" me. I told them their damn check was on the way.

I must rely on God and myself. Which one do I not trust? Where is my faith?

Dr. M. says I'm in a large flare.

5/2/89 6:30 p.m.

Today I begin Cytoxan.

I went into a rebellion yesterday afternoon. I don't want to do this. I want things to be "normal." But the reality is, I have a disease. The reality is, I must control this disease. I am not passive. I am not a martyr. I am not a "victim of" anything. I am a survivor.

Took my Cytoxan. Called Nancy first and we prayed over it, that I wouldn't throw up from it.

8:30—So far, so good. I'm shaky but okay. Already bathed (shower chair works great) and makeup on. Bed made. Dishes in dishwasher. This just might be a good day.

Hair is still shedding. I'm already grieving over it. Soon, I'll have to get a wig. Must remember to go look at wigs.

By 10 a.m. I was ready to go to the TEC.

The Texas Employment Commission Chorus

What a screwup.

I was told to wait until my name was called. By 11:15, I asked what was taking so long and I was told, "You missed your turn when the 10:00 group was called."

I told them, "I was told to wait until *my name* was called."

I finally saw a claims examiner, got chewed out because *they* didn't give me the correct printout last time—(each examiner has his favorite printout, it seems).

I am to return on the 15th with my forms all filled out, etc., etc. If I were going to get sick, it would have been then.

I left and went to Social Security. Quite a walk with my cane, but I had free parking at TEC. Social Security was confusing, to say the least.

The Social Security Symphony in C Minor, or "You're Not Sick Enough"

The nearest I could figure out was, I needed to be sick enough to have not worked for a year, was not expected to get any better or was near death, before I could qualify for a disability payment of $500 a month.

Puhleese!!!

There is something very wrong here.

The upshot is, wait and see about my unemployment. If they contest it, then I'll file for disability & SSI.

I have no pride left. I'll do what I have to do to survive.

I have $10 in cash till I get a paycheck of some kind on the 15th.

I'm definitely into fear.

5/4/89 1:00

I thought everything was all set for me to go back to work at Hampton.

But they said that since there was a break in service I had to have my case reviewed by the Board—tomorrow. They'll let me know then. Nobody can be rehired until they go through this. Could they contact my former employer and I said yes…what else could I say?

Dealt with IRS also. "We" still owe.

I don't.

Need to go to the lawyer's.

And I need to go get a handicapped-parking permit.

5/5/89 Friday p.m.

Storm kept me awake last night. Slept okay after midnight, till about 4:30 when the Darvocet wore off. I was up having coffee when my parents called about 6:30. It began okay—then went downhill.

61

I told them about the vasculitis in my left leg now.

They said they worried I may have an accident.

They kept on and on about getting someone to drive me; they don't want me to have a wreck.

I "lost it." I said *maybe that would be the best thing*, and I started to cry.

I told them I have food in the house, gas in the car, $10 in cash and $45 in the bank. No paycheck at least for 2 weeks or unemployment for 2 weeks.

Mother said they would send a check to cover my utilities, at least. I told her $70 for electric, $30 for water. Forgot the phone bill.

Dad repeated, "Get your friends to help. Call Evelyn. Have her drive you around."

What he is saying is, "I can't handle this. Get someone to take care of you."

I never thought I would be the topic of discussion in my family: "What shall we do about Marilyn?" Everybody seems to have their own idea. Terri wants to fix it with money; but in the long run, we can't continue doing that.

Mother wants to physically be here and help where they can financially.

Went to atty's office to leave note. Drove downtown for interview. Took typing test with no practice. Passed!

Took spelling test = 100%. Interviewed at Cable Connection. Stressed out over cane. What will they say/think?

They asked me to take drug test at Med/Surg clinic today.

Stopped by Sanus lab for my own blood work for Monday appt.

Went to Med Surg clinic—waited from 3:30 to 4:45 to give urine specimen.

Gave healthily—then the nurse SPILLED IT ALL.

Try again? I've never been able to "go" on command, so I must go back Monday.

Drove home in heavy 5 p.m. traffic.

This much I know: I have done more today than a well person

should. Stressed as much as possible.

But my mental attitude is okay.

I've accepted all that my illness has to give.

I also know a Great Truth:

I thought I would do God's will if He would just show me. However, I was thinking, "*I'll do God's will if He'll show me and if it fits in with my plans.*"

For instance: I told Nancy that I had always thought God wants me to have a job with insurance coverage for a preexisting illness. Sounds fine. Sounds like Hampton HMO.

But maybe part of God's plan for me is to trust Him, take a job without insurance and just pay for it myself? Who knows?

All I knew is *I've been setting limits on God.* Let Him do for me what I cannot do for myself.

He always does so much better when I stay out of His way.

5/6/89 Saturday 9:30 a.m

Legs kind of ache from all the walking yesterday.

Woke this morning crying. My father is so angry.

Then it hit me…he's not angry, really. He's *afraid.* Afraid I'll get over my head. Fear disguised as anger. "*Oh, my God, she'll get in trouble and I'll always have to take care of her and I don't know how to do that so why not just tell her whatever she's doing it's wrong so she won't do anything that I have to take care of…*"

He needs comforting, too.

5/6/89

Losses

I was walking along one day
Minding my own business
And I looked up
And I had lost my job.

It was right beside me.
It just fell off
The edge of the world
And I couldn't find it again.
I was walking along one day
Minding my own business
And I looked up
And I had lost my Health.
It was right beside me.
It was there a minute ago.
I don't know where it went.
Now, I can't get it back
And I'll never be the same again.
I was walking along one day
Minding my own business
And I looked up
And I had lost my God.
He was there a minute ago;
He was right beside me.
I don't know where He went—
But I can't seem to find Him again
I had let go of His hand
And he allowed me
To try it
On my own.
Minding my own business
Without God
Doesn't work.
I think I'll reach out my hand....
And I know He'll
Walk beside me again.

5/6/89 3:30 p.m.

Finally decided to waddle out to the mailbox—reluctantly —"Fear of Mailbox Syndrome?" Thinking Woody's picture might be there. He called this morning. Sounded down. He and his girlfriend have had a tiff. I'd call it. He said he thought it was a good picture and he wanted me to have it.

So I wasn't expecting much more than that when I brought the mail in. A letter from a creditor (of course) but it said, "let's make a deal"—a note from the city stating someone else had been chosen for the City Mgrs' secretarial job—and I remembered that man's angry eyes and said thank you, God.

A letter with no return address. Hand-written. A piece of white bond paper wrapped around a cashier's check for $100. To Marilyn Morris. From "A Friend."

Well, of course, I cried.

Then, a little informal note. No return address. Just a message—"Thinking of You" and two $5 bills fall out.

Well, I just "lost it."

I cried and cried.

Now, what do I do with all this?

Also Sanus insurance letter came…. My premium is $85.58. Coincidence?

Just God's way of remaining anonymous.

5/6/89 10:15 p.m.

Will use the $100 to pay my Sanus premium for this month. The $10 will go to gas—except Anne V. offered to fill my car up with gas on her credit card. I told her I'd let her do that and maybe tomorrow.

It is so difficult to accept help. It's just difficult accepting anything. This disease, in particular. Why? Why now? (*Why not? I hear*). And it is *now* because you can *handle* it *now*.

A year earlier, and you couldn't have done it, Marilyn. You wouldn't have built this circle of love around you. All your Sisters in Christ—your former co-workers who still keep in touch—and your family is closer to you now.

Pay the insurance for this month and keep walking.

Contact Texas Vocational Rehab for some tips…

God, there are times I feel like giving up. Completely. The struggle to keep myself alive with food, shelter, and transportation is almost getting too much for me.

Today, I can do it.

Tomorrow, who knows? I try to look on the positive side of disability and SSI.

Just think—no getting up early to hit the road to an office in all weather.

I can write all day if I want. I can have lunch with people…long lunches.

5/8/89 4 p.m.

Went to Dr. Morton, 8:30 a.m. He increased the Cytoxan to 60mg. I have lost 2 lbs. He's not concerned about that. 118 lbs.

Go back to lab and give specimen again. *This time I give copiously and this time, the girl doesn't spill it.*

On to the sub courthouse and get my handicapped parking card. I cried. Handicapped? Not me. But it will be necessary.

At home again, I went to the mailbox.

Got a card and check ($200) from Mom and Dad. For utilities and meds this month. It's more than I thought it would be.

5/9/89

Woke feeling good. Positive. Had a dream where a door opened and there were all these options.

I felt good about it.

Talked to Terri last night. She wants me to call *her* when I'm "down," not Mom and Dad. She said she didn't want me to tell her I'm "fine" when I'm not.

I apologized.

She said get rid of the house. I agreed. It's no sin. She wants me to make a budget without a house payment and see if she sends $100 every two weeks for the next couple of months.

66

Would that help? She's willing to do that.

I told her yes, I'd do that, and it would help. And thank you. Feel like I lost today.

5/10/89

If you hear it from enough people, it must be so. "Go file for SSI." That would be best. Then I could just work a little bit to supplement the $400 SSI—up to $2,000 per month? Have to check on that. And I'd get medicine.

Feeling "urgency" today to get all this pulled together and get on with it. With what? Getting a job? I'm going to check into some of the lower paying jobs, which would be less stressful.

Sanus won't pay for prescription meds. Sounds like I need Medicaid.

Things are not going my way. I'm feeling rebellious again. Every suggestion is met with heel digging.

Lord, I don't want to feel this way. I want to get on with it.

5/15/89 3 a.m.

Up again. Can't sleep. Went to Boerne on Friday with Bob and family. We left here around 8 p.m. Got there at 1:30 a.m. Went straight to sleep. I took a Restoil since I knew I would be too tired to sleep.

Woke Sat. to the aroma of Mom's pancakes, coffee, juice, grapefruit and coffee. Felt really helpless, not getting around. I found it a bit difficult going up and down the stairs, but everybody helped.

Went into the Sr. Citizen's Center and got introduced as "My daughter with lupus." Those were the women on Mom's Walk to Amaeus who know and love my mother and who have been praying for me. I felt it and thanked them and told them it helped me a lot.

I napped that afternoon. Wonderful breeze. Didn't want to get up.

We put a roast in the oven before we left for church and it was done when we got back.

When we left, I hugged Mom and told her I loved her. And when I got in the car, Dad came over and leaned in and hugged me hard and said, "I love you." I told him I was glad we could talk. What a blessing.

The trip home was kinda noisy with all 3 girls whining. I had more trouble with my vision, too; I told Bob I was glad he was driving and not me, because I *couldn't see big road signs until we were right on them. My bladder drove me crazy, too; had to stop about every 10 minutes.* I told Bob, "I need to stop now. I mean now." At a service station in Marble Falls, I couldn't get my jumpsuit down fast enough and peed all over myself and all over the floor.

I felt like a big baby, asking Bob and Evelyn to open the trunk so I could get dry underwear and jeans. My shoes had to come off, too; in fact, I threw them away.

Arrived home, ate, read the paper, took a couple of calls and tried to sleep. Even with a Restoil, I can't sleep.

So thirsty. I fixed Gatorade, black cherry juice, cranapple juice —peed every ½ hour. I had no more to drink either. Must remember to tell the doctor.

5/16/89 8:30 a.m.

Taking it real easy today. Yesterday was too damn much. Didn't sleep Sunday evening.

My legs shake.

Went to Dr. Larson for this bladder problem. It is an infection. Got a prescript for Septra. Should clear it right up.

Also asked about vision—blurry...referred to a Dr. Zachary. But Sanus won't do that. Need to call for a referral to an optometrist. Cost about $30 altogether.

But I have to have my vision improve. My vision is real blurry.

Is it lupus? Or is it just time to have my prescription changed? I hope I can stay out of that fear.

Gibraltar called with some kind of "deal" that I don't

understand. What I think she's saying is we can work out with the lien holders and a realtor and while I wouldn't get any money out of it, I'd be out from under the payments.

Waiting for my unemployment to start in ten days. Need to pay a few bills. Call electric co.

Then to Bombay Co for an interview. Not a good one, either.

She asked about my cane. I told her I had vasculitis and was being treated for it. And it wouldn't hurt my job performance. Nevertheless, I knew I was "out."

Got a letter from Hampton Hospital Corp. I had not been selected to join the temp pool.

I think they are shitheads. I want them to tell me why they can't use me.

I know it's because of lupus.

Maybe I'm just supposed to let the federal government take care of my needs. If they can place me in a handicapped stress-free job, that's what I'll need.

Woody sent $50 yesterday. Bless him.

Rain, thunder, and lightning. Good napping weather.

5/16/89

Storms

Storms on the outside
Making storms on my inside.

Rage flows through me
As the wind howls
Through the trees.
I weep as the rain
Pounds the earth
Both the rain
And my tears
Are cleansing.

But what pain we must feel
To receive that cleansing!
As the rain nourishes some areas,
It wreaks havoc in others.
I am powerless
Over the seasons
And their accompanying changes.
I am powerless
Over my disease
And its accompanying changes.
I grieve for my former self
Who could cram 36 hours into 24.
Who could walk briskly.
Whose handwriting
Was not laborious
But spontaneous.
Grieving is normal,
They tell me.
It will diminish,
In time,
Like the spring storm
That passes over me.

5/17/89 2 a.m.

A thought occurred to me in these early morning hours: "*You are setting limits on God again. Marilyn, you think you have to have a government job? Well, maybe not. Just keep walking.*"

A tiny voice beside me says, "*I'm tired of walking. I'm tired of waiting. I'm just tired, dear God. Help me. Heal me now.*"

I must stop my ideas of what job I need. Nothing has happened yet.

5/19/89 6:30 p.m.

Almost too tired to write. Shitty day. Started off with a call from Mom and Dad. I told them I was very tired. Cried.

They couldn't handle it. Dad "had to go." I told Mom I knew he couldn't understand my disease. She knows, too.

Cried some more.

Was late for my appt. at Catholic Charities. At 9:30 was told to come back at 1:00 p.m. Stopped by the lab to have lab work done for Dr. Morton's appt. Monday.

Left there and came home for lunch. Couldn't get left contact out. Boo-hooed and then went to TSO to get them to take it out.

Surprise! They looked and said it wasn't there!

I must have lost it at the lab or at Catholic Charities. I think I have insurance on it, so it's okay.

Back to Catholic Charities by 1 p.m. Some boy who looked all of thirteen asked me a lot of questions, took my Social Security card and driver's license number and statement of disability and finally decided they would pay my electric bill.

Just this once.

Then he mentions a food voucher. I took it. Went to the specified market and got $30 worth of food: a roast, hamburger, canned veg and fruit, etc., 5 lb potatoes, lettuce, 3 tomatoes, hamburger buns.

By now it was 2:30 and I was worn out. Came home and put food up and crashed on the couch. Totally exhausted. Also have a little stomachache. Can't imagine why.

Just feel so frustrated. My eyesight is awful. I need to have my lens changed but must wait for the Sanus voucher before I can have it done.

Interesting thought: *How am I going to get the money to move if I can't sell the house or go to work?* I'll have to get a job first—can't depend on UI for that. Must earn more than $840 mo.

Gibraltar should send that info soon. Then I can move—provided I have a job—and get on with my life. Not that I haven't been "working." I have worn myself out.

It never seems enough. My body tells me it's enough. I'm learning to listen to my body and not feel guilty. At least, not too guilty.

God, I had a bad day today. I am so tired. Everything seems to be too much trouble.

But—I've made it through another day.

5/21/89 12:20 a.m.

Couldn't write in this journal until now. Overwhelming day. Started out at 7 a.m. I put my column on the computer and was ready to go when Nancy called around noon. We had planned to have lunch at Denny's and did. She came to get me. I couldn't eat all my omelet so got a doggie bag.

We left it at Nancy's while we dropped off my column and stopped to pick up the grab bar for the tub.

I owe her so much. I don't know what I would do without her. She gave me a huge chunk of magnolia and even put it in water in the blue vase when we got home.

We put the grab bar where I will reach it from the commode, too.

Jimmie had said she would be at Sam's and would get me some Gatorade. Wow, did she. A gallon jar. Plus—a box full of canned goods and baggies of chicken strips, mozzarella rolls, flautas, and more. I was just overwhelmed.

Got my check Saturday, too, so that helps. I'll start on my bills tomorrow. Everybody will get something—even if it's just $5.

God, what is this disease doing to me?

This disease has changed my handwriting; it has caused changes in my skin and I have a moon face, and by God, I'm angry.

I spend my time putting out brushfires.

I don't want to obsess over this disease. My friends are probably tired of this disease, too. They want to help and make it go away, but they are also powerless.

5/22/89

Weight. 110

Dry mouth; meds same; *I now have Sjogren's Syndrome*—dry eyes, dry mouth. Need to use—ugh, it even *sounds* yucky—artificial saliva...

Another Damn Disease!

5/23/89 11:30 p.m.

I found out today I have *diabetes*, too. That explains all the bladder problems and vision problems. I'm taking medication for the diabetes now, too.

On the way home, I said out loud, in my car, "*Okay, God, so now I have another damn disease! If you've got anything else for me, why don't you give it to me right now, instead of stringing it out?*"

Fear overwhelms me when I think of my financial situation. What am I going to do? I need to work; yet I can't. It's all I can do some days to just stand up. I'm going to fall, or have an accident, or something awful like that.

5/23/89

This diabetes is just another event to cope with. Another change in lifestyle.

My eyesight should clear up now.

I just would like to be able to *walk better.* Dr. Morton said the vasculitis is a little better, but I can't tell, I still fall a lot.

Losing 8 lbs in two weeks didn't help me. Nothing tastes good. Cottonmouth driving me nuts.

Must sit down and pay bills today.

Feel guilty that I'm not dressing for work. But I'm not supposed to do that today.

Today, I'll just take care of things around here...and I'll nurture myself.

5/25/89 2 p.m.

I woke up grieving.

God, I am so alone.

I am 51 years old. I have a crappy disease that does awful things to my body. My personal appearance is changing. I am losing my hair. I was so proud of my thick hair. It is getting gray even as it falls out.

I can't walk well. I lurch. I am tired most of the time and can't cope with housework for fear of falling, or hurting myself.

I was so independent, and now I must depend on others.

I have no income other than UI and my family.

Nobody has a job for me and SS and Disability take forever.

I hear from everybody: "Why don't you...?" in a friendly tone, helpful, loving, even, and yet I hear an edge of criticism to it, or "Why haven't you done that already?"

In short, I feel defensive. I *am* doing all I can. I *am* looking for a job. I *am* following my doctor's orders. I *am busy* all the time, either going to an interview or "settling things" that never seem to work out, such as the lawsuit.

My friends are wonderful. They have literally kept me alive.

But my friends can also almost kill me with their "helpfulness."

They don't understand: "Echinacea builds up your immune system. Here, take some."

I told my friend my immune system is on overdrive and I don't need it built up, thank you. But she didn't understand. It was supposed to be good for a person.

I had a cold one day—rather, several days, and I was advised to take echinacea. Ordered, almost. When I stalled, somehow intuitively knowing it would be bad for me, my friend came to my house, rang the bell, and when I opened the door, thrust a plastic bag of pills at me:

"Take these. I want you to get better."

It's hard to explain to your friends that you can't take what *they* take. Another reason for feeling "different" from others.

God, here's a list. A kind of comparison of benefits...the bad stuff on one side, the good on the other. Help me find the balance!

I hate to hear: "But you look wonderful" when I feel so bad.

Laugh. Love it. Tell the person "Thank you, but I have an *inside disease.*" or, "The fever gives me a glow."

Housework is a bitch.

Break it up into small pieces; accept offers of help.

Moving to an apartment will be stressful...

You'll have help.

Giving up my house will be traumatic.

Not really. The house is too much for you now.

Sleep is disturbed.

You won't die from it.

I have blurry vision.

It'll clear up.

I lost my contact lens...

So what? Wear your glasses, or get out an old lens.

You've spent too much money.

How much is too much? I have to eat!

I feel like a child.

That's okay. You are a child. God's child.

I feel rebellious.

Go ahead and rebel. You couldn't do it as a child.

I feel angry at myself for not doing "right."

By whose standards?

This disease won't go away.

It won't, but you can put it to sleep for a long time.

I have lupus, vasculitis, and diabetes.

I am handling all of this as well as I can.

I can't move around very well.

At least I can still walk.

I am alone.

It's probably best right now.
I am 51 years old.
So what?
My hair is coming out.
It looks fine now. Get a wig later.
I have no income. That's not right.
I have UI and applied for SSI, etc.
I'm not doing enough....
I'm doing all I can each day.
I feel ignorant.
I'm learning.
I've been fired three times! It doesn't look good on my resume...
All were due to my disease.
I feel like a cloud has settled over me that says, "Don't hire her. She has a disease."
These people are ignorant.
I feel overwhelmed.
You're *whelmed*, but not overly so.
I feel like I have to complete my lists each day.
Don't follow them.
I feel I am no good to anybody.
Bullshit. People depend on me.
I receive too much "advice."
Sort it out; some of it may be valid.
I don't have a way to "explain" my disease.
Find one; a condensed version that others can understand.

I've come to realize that life does hurt. One way or another. We "choose our own pain"—stay or go? Hold on or let go? Love or not love? Risk or play it safe?

I also know today that I have anger as my companion. I don't know how to deal with anger. I have denied it all my life, stuffed it down, and now it demands to be set loose.

I truly believe my physical pain would be lessened if I could rid myself of this anger—this rage.

And what am I angry about?

Everything and nothing. Everybody and nobody.

Just keep walking.

One bright spot about The Cane:

My youngest niece, Stephanie, is fascinated by my closet full of clothes; she plays dress-up every time she comes over. Parades in front of us in high heels (which I can no longer wear) and long dresses, hats, purses and "joolery."

When she sees my cane, she is fascinated. Adds that to her fashion show. Along with my newly purchased wig, which I reluctantly remove, revealing my patchy scalp.

Then she utters the line…"*For Christmas, I want a wig and a cane…*"

I don't know whether to laugh or cry.

So I do both.

I must believe in myself: that I am capable, competent and worthwhile just as a person.

God, I don't know why I'm going through this disease. You do. I feel that I am becoming "softer" somehow. More responding to you and others. Willing to share my feelings, thoughts, and experiences.

I feel a certain amount of serenity, knowing things are really in Your hands. Maybe in my childhood I put my father as my God. I depended on him and tried to please him by being a good girl and making good grades. So he would not go off again and abandon me. And of course, he did—or I felt he did.

My earthly father is not my God. There is only one God, and He loves me unconditionally and I don't have to do anything to please Him. Just be the woman He wants me to be. He will never abandon me, even though it seems He has. I must not think, well, God is off somewhere doing something great for me and He'll be back soon.

And I'll just have to wait and be a good girl and work hard so when He does return I can tell him how good I have been and how busy I have been and then I'll be rewarded by my father's presence. For a while…then it starts again.

God doesn't leave me to do His will for me. He doesn't "come and go." His presence is always with me. I just haven't recognized it.

God is always with me. He fixes things. I am enough for him. He created me, and He is pleased with me. Always.

I can go to movies when they're not crowded. I can take a nap after lunch. I can stay up as late as I want. I can go back to school, if possible. I can spend more time on my spiritual growth and help others do the same.

But oh, how I wish I didn't have to live by myself. (Notice I didn't say, "Go through this by myself.") I have so many supportive friends—who help me through my days, but it would be so nice to have a companion with me in the night. To be here with me for dinner and conversation or quiet reading together, or even a fight or two to keep things lively.

Some readings ask if I want to be healed? The answer is *Yes.* I want my former health restored. I want to work. I don't like this disease and the slow, painful progress. The major organ involvement has evidently started.

As long as I don't hurt in the joints, I am pretty darn cocky. As long as I am able to bring home a paycheck, I deny the *reality* of this disease.

But when I ended up hospitalized, was fired and had no funds in sight, all the pride left me. I must face the reality that I might never be able to work again. To provide for myself.

It is truly humbling to walk awkwardly with a cane. To stumble through the house, holding on to furniture. To know—in your gut—that people don't want you to work there because you're costing them too much money with your illness.

The bottom line is *the bottom line. (Nothing personal.)*

Life Is a Temporary Assignment

I will always appreciate the temporary company who took a chance on me when I lurched into their offices, carrying a cane, and signed up as a temp.

I was sent to a bank, where I showed up every morning for two weeks, stepping carefully across the polished marble floor, doing what I had to do, and finally, making it across the lobby without falling flat on my face.

My coworkers never said a word about it, either.

Shitty day. Started out to take the census test. Couldn't take it...they are "full." I was ticked.

Went to TU Electric and dropped off my voucher from Catholic Charities. Then put bills in main post office box. Went to another temp company and signed up for employment. Also TCOM; they told me to come back and take a typing and spelling test after lunch.

I have to do that tomorrow.

Went to lupus group tonight. Found out that I'm doing pretty good, after all. Need to cut out caffeine. It's a vaso-constrictor. Have a bit of pleurisy, too, due to weather.

5/26/89 6:50 a.m.

Yesterday I fell in the hallway. Was wearing a small heel. Left leg turned and I toppled over against the tray holding the silver tea set.

Scared the hell out of me.

Then I went to TCOM to take my typing test. Flunked twice. Get to go back and take it twice, though.

Came home feeling yucky. Lay down. I stopped by and got stamps and a book on disability at Half Price Books. It's excellent. I plan to use my little red microwave cart to push around the house...kinda lean on it....

My folks called.

I told them about the diabetes. They were surprised. I asked Dad about it. He said no sugar, carbs. Eat fruits and veg. And eat an orange if you get shaky.

5/26/89 7 a.m.

I called to get some counseling. I'm carrying too many burdens. Can't sort things out. Disease, medications…all combine to assault me. I need a balance. I need to be able to cope rationally.

I don't like what I'm having to do. I want someone else to do it…make the calls, give me the information. I get confused, fragmented, disoriented—too much information is bombarding me. "Why don't you—have you tried? Etc. Plus "helpful hints" for my disease.

Yet I know it's all well meaning.

5/27/89 6:30 a.m.

Dying Is the Easy Part

I have finally realized what *chronic* means. It will not go away. I knew that in my head. Today I just know it in my gut.
I am still feeling overwhelmed by all that's going on with me. The disability stuff, moving, my being so slow getting around. I need to remember to stress capability, not disability.
Barbara, Nancy and Liz have ganged up on me. They have each told me they thought there was a time there when I didn't want to live.
They were right.
Some days I feel that way.
But today I have a goal.

5/28/89 Sunday 7:30 a.m.

I had such a good day yesterday. I cleaned house. Even vacuumed.

Rested in between cleanings. Feel a sense of accomplishment. That I have my environment under control.

Talked to Carmen a long time. She also said she thought for a while I

80

had chosen death instead of life. I don't know when the turning point came, except I just got angry and decided to let that anger work for me.

I don't know what will happen next. Today I have $5 in my purse. Today, I'm not in total fear. Today, I will let God guide me. Today, I'm at peace.

And that scares me!

5/29/89

Woke feeling sad. Could be that is because I babysat Katie, Stephanie and Jessie last night—and I fixed spaghetti and missed my kids and realized I may never have grandchildren.

Could be it's just my meds ganging up on me, too.

My hair continues to fall out. That's depressing.

God has a job for me, in His time.

Today, I am okay. I have food, gas, and shelter. I have some mobility left. Some energy.

I am capable. In the name of Jesus, I rebuke the demons that tie me down.

5/30/89

I now believe in angels and demons. *This Present Darkness* is snaring me in a way. But I know that evil can snare us one way or another, so why not personify evil?

Found out lots of stuff re: fed jobs...by phone. GSA, TEC Vocational Rehab. Are all supposed to be direct hire. Will go to TEC tomorrow and fill out their cards.

5/31/89 5:50 a.m.

Today, I start taking Micronase. 2 at 2x a day. I am in fear about that. At least until I talk to Dr. Morton. Will pick up the lab slip this a.m. and go to TEC for Federal job listings.

I am in such a grief process. I am losing my house. My income is almost nil. Really crappy day. But I got into expectations. And I can't expect anything.

Lawyer called. They will serve Doug with papers soon.
Good.
But I'm afraid of facing him in court.

6/4/89 Sunday

I am tired and frustrated.

Dad doesn't know how to treat me anymore. He either hovers or is distant. Mom is almost the same way. They just don't know what to do with me now.

I need to tell them more often—I need to tell Mom "I can do this" or "I need help with this…" don't let them guess.

Oh, God. Help me to know you have not abandoned me. Keep me out of this awful pit.

6/5/89

Wt. 114
Diabetes
Micronase added Increase Cytoxan to 100 mg
Foot drop still….

6/5/89 5 a.m.

Went to bed at 8:30 last night. Woody called and I cried when I hung up. He called right back. Afraid for my crying. I told him I'll be okay…it's just that I am so tired…physically and emotionally.

Sometimes I just have to cry.

I'm grieving my past life. For all the things I thought I needed —really, wanted—and it hurts to give things up. But things are just that. Ideas are painful to give up…the idea that I am someone other than who I am…I always thought I was such a proud person independent, sassy, even vengeful. Able to take care of myself. And brittle.

Now I'm finding out I can't be that way anymore. I must depend on others. I must give up some things. I'll have a garage sale, move to an apartment. The house is just a house. I'll make a new home for myself. Heaven knows I've done that before.

But first I have to grieve. And that takes a long time. I was supposed to go to counseling today, but it was postponed till next Monday. I'm sure professional help will benefit me.

I swing out of one mood into another. Pessimism to optimism. It's partly the meds.

Fear has had control of me all my life. It's time to acknowledge it and get on with living free. I can't wait to get out of this place, truly. It has become a burden to me. Seemingly, life has become a burden to me...but I can't dwell on that negative thought.

Nobody has an easy life. It just looks that way to me. I was such a princess all my life. Now I'm having to find out who I really am.

6/6/89

Well, TEC finally came through. $630 arrived in one check. Plus Woody sent $25. I was so tired and discouraged and could see only my problems. All of them at once

I am just now realizing the dreadful power of this lupus. It has wreaked havoc in my life and I'm angry. The things it could do to me further infuriates me...I could have more major organ involvement. I could go blind—have seizures—no telling!

I pray for health, for a job, for a place to live.

I pray for all those dear to me, and for my enemies.

I pray to live through this day.

6/9/89

I need people. I realize. I've been almost isolating. It's easy to do. But I know I'm better off among people, most of the time.

Am going to the Women's Center this a.m. and check out the

83

job leads. Diane C is there—maybe we can find me a piddly little job. Dear God, guide me in the direction I need to go.

6/9/89 6:45 p.m.

Diane was of "some help." Suggested I go back to Hampton and ask if it was insurance problem or something I said or did...or didn't say or do. I should tell them that since I have my own insurance they don't need to insure me.

I would have to have the courage to confront those people and I'm not sure I could do that.

Nancy and I went to look at a wig. Not only did we look but also I got one!

It looks natural—feels good—price was right: $55 altogether, styling, incl. She had to cut it a lot, closer to my own hairstyle. Finished there about 4 p.m.

Mood is a little better today. Probably because nearly everything went my way. Tonight I'm looking forward to just being a couch potato in front of the TV.

Too bad I can't read the program.

6/11/89 p.m.

It's Dad's birthday. I called him and wished him a happy 70th. It's hard for me to believe my childhood young prince is now an old man. But that is reality. *He never really was a prince. Only in my fantasy.*

Got some half-moon reading glasses today and they work. And some hats.

Hats

One straw hat
Started it all.
A fun thing to have,
To wear with a flair.
On hat led to another
And then there were three.
Might as well discover
What others there might be.
Wal-Mart has dozens
And the price was right, too.
I picked up "several"
Red, yellow, and blue
And black, and another straw hat
And did I have fun!
Almost like playing dress-up
I thought I'd never be done.
I wore my blue hat today…
I must say I looked chic.
It gave my spirits a lift
Compliments I didn't seek.
But I got them, anyway,
And it made me feel just great.
Thank you, Lord,
For little things—
Like blue straw hats
And a sunny day
And the courage to face my infirmities
With grace and humor and strength.

6/12/89 a.m.

Took the phone off the hook early this a.m. Rain and thunder and lightning. No TV. Have resentment against the cable company. Every time it storms, it goes out.

Today I will go to City Hall, TEC, Waterworks and counseling. It's probably too much, but it's necessary.

It looks like the diabetes may be under control. The vasculitis a bit better. I am also grateful that today, I don't have to be out driving to work in all this rain.

And to a job I really didn't like.

I told everybody I liked it, but it was repetitive and I never felt comfortable with it. "Over supervised," Policy and Procedure kept changing.

I know there is no ideal job. I don't know what signs to look for when considering a job, either.

Except for the man with the angry eyes.

I need to trust my instincts more.

6/12/89 p.m.

Went to City Hall and applied for legal secretary job. Have to take a typing test Friday.

Then on to counseling. It was inconclusive, I think.

I just vibrated and cried and told him about my illness. I am doing all I can. The rest is up to God.

The church counselor also encouraged me to confront Hampton. Tell them that as long as I have my own insurance, why can't they hire me back? I know I have had good reviews. All I need is courage: "Courage to change the things I can…"

6/14/89 10 p.m.

I have had 5 good days in a row. Can't believe it. Even bought some gold shrimp earrings tonight at Foley's...

I'm worth it.

6/14/89

Went to see Hampton Hospital execs today. Left a note telling I had my own insurance, etc. If they respond, fine. If not, maybe I should just leave it alone.

But I'm glad I took the action and was willing to confront for the first time in my life. No matter what the outcome. I did it for me.

God, I feel you are preparing me for a job. I am being made stronger each day.

6/15/89

Totally frustrated this morning. Went to Fed. Bldg. To see who would do direct hire. Everyone looked at me blankly. No leads. Lots of walking.

Felt good most of the day. *Six days in a row.* Thank you, God.

6/20/89 a.m.

I am feeling overwhelmed again. And fearful. I'm afraid I won't get a job. I'm afraid I won't have any insurance. I'm afraid I won't survive.

I'm afraid of myself.

I'm afraid that if I don't get a job soon, before unemployment insurance runs out, I will commit suicide.

Those thoughts have entered my mind. I don't want to, but there seems to be no way out...Just die and get all this mess over with.

Life has been so tedious at times. I know it's wrong thinking wanting things to go smoothly all the time. But I don't see, dear God, why I am

having to go through this. Are you testing me?
It seems I've struggled so long. I'm so tired of my life being so difficult.

6/23/89 7 a.m.

Attorney had bad news about the mortgage. We can't take Mom and Dad off. I went home in total terror. Crying.

Called Realtor Mark Gregory to put the house up for sale. Might as well try. I don't understand why Gibraltar would rather have the house back—or leave it unoccupied, rather than refinance.

I couldn't cope with anything more yesterday. I cancelled my appts with the other agencies and took a nap. Also slept well last night.

I'm emotionally exhausted. Heartache. Stressed.

I feel like my parents will be angry with me. I'm a scared little kid who can't tell her mother and father that she has done something "bad." Then they will be angry with me and abandon me. But these are old tapes.

6/26/89 Monday

The folks have come and gone. I was different this time. I told them my lawyer said we can't get their names off my mortgage, and they didn't have a stroke, or yell, or say anything else except "Oh."

I'm trying not to make money my God today.

6/27/89 Thursday 1 a.m.

I received in the mail an American Express money order for $100. Plus $10 in cash. Anonymous, of course.

My publisher at the newspaper called and said if I could deliver next week's column on Wednesday, she'd give me my check early.

The realtor and his wife came by to appraise the house and sign a contract. He noticed my Al-Anon literature and asked me about my religion.

I sidestepped and said I was more spiritual than religious, and I said, "I know God sells houses."

He then told me of his experiences in seeing the sick healed. Said he had been praying for me and would work with me any way he could. And before they left, we stood and held hands and prayed.

Rather, they prayed.

I blubbered.

God certainly brings people into our lives just when we need them.

7/1/89 Saturday

Got a call from the temporary company. They have an assignment for me starting Monday for 2 weeks.

I don't know Microsoft but they assure me that I can do it.

I'm apprehensive about going back to work. Will I have the energy? Can I cope with the stress?

Will they like me? says the little kid.

Laugh for the day: I make too much money to qualify for food stamps. $626 is the max for one person per month.

7/2/89 Sunday p.m.

I like to hear the thunder...if it's far away. Bad storm tonight. Wind and rain and thunder and lightning. But I wasn't afraid. Haven't been for about 2-3 years now.

I'm more afraid of going to work tomorrow. For the first time in 3 months.

7/4/89 Tuesday

No plans for today. What do people like me do on a holiday dedicated to sun and water and sports? When I'm feeling so crummy and crippled? Yet I don't want to stay here by myself. What alternatives? A movie? Shopping? Both cost money. And it's so hot. Not good for me.

I recognized fear yesterday at work. I'm afraid of anybody in authority. Even on a temp. basis. Men, especially. Then, when I realize I'm afraid, I swing the other way, and become sassy and cocky and brittle. I need the balance that other people have. A little respect for authority, but not fear. A little independence but not isolation.

My survival does not depend on another person.

7/16/89 Monday a.m.

An exercise in futility. That's the way I feel this morning about "looking for a job." It seems so useless. I am in a negative mood. Looking for work is stressful. So is being unemployed. I have an appt. Friday with Vocational Rehab. Hope they can untangle some of the bureaucratic red tape.

God, will this never end? This time of uncertainty. This time of self-doubt and indecision.

There is so much to do and only so much time. Only so much energy. Only so much of me. I feel ready to explode, sometimes, out of sheer frustration. Well-wishers drive me crazy. I'm doing all I can for myself, yet it appears it's not enough. Yet I can't say that. I have the temp jobs…but penalized by TEC for working. You can't win.

On Lupus

Lupus is a crappy disease.
It sneaks up on my blind side
And assaults me when
I'm not paying attention.
Just when I think
Things are going well,
A new problem appears
To give me hell.
Vasculitis followed the
Pneumonia bit.
I lost my job,
Acquired a cane.
And then diabetes hit.
Medicine and pills
And shots and
Watching my diet.
Is that all there is
To life?
I walk funny now.
Even with my cane.
My hair is still
Coming out.
My vision is changing
And I can't keep a contact lens in my eye.
My face is blown up
Like a balloon,
In that famous
"Moon Face" form.
Weight gain,
Bloating and ankles swell.
Oh, but you're not in pain today,
Baby girl.
Be grateful for a day
Free of pain.
Remember what it was like—
Pre-Plaquenil
And Prednisone!

91

8/7/89

Spirituality vs. Religiosity

My realtor and his wife invited me to a healing service the next Sunday—at a charismatic church.

Well, I'm Episcopalian, and was hesitant, but I figured, what did I have to lose?

These people spoke in tongues. They waved their arms and danced around.

God, I breathed, please don't let me get up there and faint and flap around like I've seen them do on TV.

And then the service was over and everyone was leaving.

All but us.

An elder of the church approached me and asked, "Do you want to be healed?"

I nodded and he led me to the front of the church, where no one was paying the least bit of attention to me.

Good.

He showed me passages in the Bible that told of healing miracles and asked if I believed.

I nodded again.

He asked us to pray and then he took a vial of oil from his pocket and made the sign of the cross on my forehead.

Well, this Episcopalian lost it.

I bawled and squalled, and I don't cry pretty.

But I didn't fall down and flop around.

He then told me that I might not be healed right now. It may be next week. It may be next month or next year, and I might want to come back again, but, he assured me, "You will be healed."

We left and went to lunch and they took me home and about two weeks later I noticed I didn't have to use my cane.

8/28/89 1:40 a.m.

Oh, Mary Kay! What You've Done to Me

I signed my contract to be a Mary Kay counselor on 8/23.
Made my first sale on 8/24.

Am I doing the right thing? Who knows? All I know is I have
to give it my best shot. If I don't I'll always wonder. And just
think—I've already made my first sale.

9/11/89 Monday a.m.

I'm tired of fighting life. I'm tired of taking medicine that
doesn't seem to do a hell of a lot of good.

I'm tired of fighting government bureaucracy, of filling out
forms, of "justifying my existence."

I'm tired of people giving me advice.

I'm tired of people asking me if I have a job yet.

I'm tired of people asking me how I feel.

I'm tired of feeling like a criminal because I'm ill.

I'm tired of this disease.

What more can I do? My therapist assures me that I'm doing
everything humanly possible to help myself survive. Yet it seems
useless. Nothing is happening. I'm running into brick walls. What
are my options?

Give up and live on disability—if it comes through. That
seems appealing at times. Just sit back and let "somebody" take
care of me.

Get a job...any job...to keep money coming in...just to keep
the house, etc., and then when I get sick again, get fired again, file
for unemployment again and start the same shitty cycle all over
again.

Continue to work temporary and draw unemployment until
something comes through with the state or county. Go along

with them and Dad's proposal to keep the house for now and then try to sell the house later.

I feel like a kid who is being told she's a "bad girl." I'm not. I have a chronic illness that prevents me from working and earning enough to keep this house. Period.

Now, either I accept monetary help from Mom and Dad (so they won't have to put a lien on their property) and Terri (who has been sending money all along) or I just give up, move to an apt. and let a foreclosure go through—and ruin Mom and Dad's credit.

And try to get my disability…. Which may or may not be approved.

It's too much, God.

I'm tired of it all.

9/15/89 Friday a.m.

Called in sick this morning. Had an assignment with the temp company, just for today. Felt queasy and had diarrhea last night…so decided, screw it this morning and am still in bed. Headache and backache the worst. *I have to remember I have lupus.* When the weather changes, I get sick at my stomach.

I also have to remember not to beat up on myself. "Normal" people get sick, too. So whether it's lupus-induced, or weather (virus) induced, I'm feeling crummy today and I get to stay home—in bed—and take care of myself. What a luxury. The old me would have struggled up and gone to work and made myself worse. Instead I'm lying in bed, drinking tea and feeling okay about it.

My counselor at Family Services, Marjorie, can be credited with this new change. She is so encouraging. It occurred to me when we were talking bout SSI, etc., that if I do go on it, it won't have to permanent…just a "pause."

I told her that I pictured myself as giving up, defeated, if I took SSI.

She then said, "Not at all. It could be just a rest. A time to regroup. Get yourself well in mind, body and spirit…. Then you can go on."

"Oh," I said. (Boing!)

Also brought to light the revelation that I no longer have to prove anything to Doug. Or to anybody. I will no longer live my life according to other people's expectations.

I feel that now. Knew it in my head before, but now I feel it in my gut.

It's hard to get rid of all the old "shoulds and oughts." She has encouraged me to keep up with Mary Kay as it seems to be liberating me.

Sold $198 of Mary Kay product last night.

What am I learning about myself?

I'm okay, just as I am. Chronic illness is part of me, but I am not my illness. Not all things can be attributed to lupus, either.

11/10/89 Friday 10 p.m.

Another dream last night. I am driving into a parking garage. It is icy. Other cars are trying to enter the garage. Their drivers get out and push their cars up. I wonder if I can do the same. I must stand back, out of their way, lest they slide backwards and hit me. I look at the ice: it is mushy so I can do it. I can push my car up the ramp.

Lupus II

Lupus is a fear,
A very real fear.
It hides in my body
Silent, for the most part.
Reminding me of its presence
Occasionally with an ache here,
A twinge, there.
Most of the time
Lupus and I co-exist.
It is an uneasy truce, however.

I fear lupus is secretly stockpiling
Nuclear weapons,
And Lupus is afraid
That I will find a way
To win this devastating war
Without firing a shot.
So there.
If guts, determination and faith,
And hope and prayer
Could be scientifically measured,
There would be a
Richter scale of ten plus
Riding on this disease.
But in the alternative,
I take my medications,
And obey my doctor's instructions
As to laboratory tests,
And no high heels,
(Vanity, vanity! But, hey,
I'm still a female!)
And try to lose weight now.
Be gentle on yourself,
A bit at a time,
And report any chills or fever.
Well, that's all well and good.
My body is doing pretty good...
It's my emotions that are
Running amok.
I'm old.
I'm unattractive.
I'm fat.
I'm sick.
I'm poor.
The devil really
Got hold of me.
I can't do anything

About my age.
I'm old—well,
I'm old—er. Better.
I'm unattractive?
Not true. I look good.
Everybody says so.
I take great care
To look good.
I'm fat?
Overweight, for sure.
I can lose it.
I'm sick.
Nothing can be done about that.
I'm poor—relatively speaking.
I hate it.
But I can do something about it.
I am doing something about it.

11/29/89

Am I supposed to just "survive" and not have any goals? Nothing to strive for, no aim or purpose, other than just to get through the day? One day after another? Can't I dream? Can't I plan?

I am so angry that this disease has robbed me of my plans. Never to know how I'll feel—what my health may be like—Christmas preparations have me "spinning"—what if? Well, what if? Christmas will still be here whether I am ready or not.

I'm feeling sorrow—grief—for my former self—my health—I want to tune out.

12/18/89

Shingle Bells, Shingle Bells....

As if lupus, diabetes and vasculitis weren't enough...I get the shingles, an affliction that I would suffer sporadically for the next few years. Pain on top of pain.

1/1/90

A New Year.
Why don't I feel joyous?
Why don't I have happy anticipation of the year before me?
As I look back on the year gone by
I can see all my problems
And their solutions.
I know that God held me in His arms then
But I'm not so sure He'll do it again.

1/21/90

In a lot of pain. Worried about the hurting in my lungs. Am I getting sick again?

Life is tough. I don't want to keep looking for a job. God, where is my job? What am I supposed to do?

2/26/90 Sunday p.m.

Weekend was okay...bought jeans and shorts and tops...bigger sizes. Pissed off. Dr. said last week to increase the Pred instead of continuing to decrease.

I don't want to get sick again, so I'll *have* to increase the med. Costs a bunch since Sanus doesn't have my new card yet, showing I have met the deductible.

Isn't it interesting? I know today I don't have to look for anything with my coworkers. Great. (I am at a bank now.) One of the bosses is taking me to lunch to show his appreciation for the work I've done. Period. Philip gave me candy for the same reason. People do those things just because.

Every day I'll pray: Thank you, God, for my perfect job. Thank you, God, for my perfect health.

As if I already had them.

My health is better.

Today I have a job.

5/28/90 Memorial Day

Am astounded that I haven't written in my journal since Feb. Why: Too busy? Too scared?

What has transpired since Feb?

The Bank Job:

I plunged into my work, and one day I was replacing the CEO's secretary for two weeks. That sent me into total terror, but when that bank went bankrupt, I was the one who was called back for a year's assignment, and then I stayed and worked for the trustee.

Well, I'm still at the bank. The old bosses are out. Trustee came. Everything okay with that.

Asked for and got benefits. Raise is coming.

Dr. visit last week. Blood work looks good. Will check next month to see if the adrenal glands are working yet. Then I can start getting off the Pred. And up the Imuran.

My hair is coming back in, curly and thick. I can walk. I feel very good—still tired a lot, but I do a lot.

Lupe, say your prayers! She seems to be in a coma—or at least in a deep sleep.

Shhh. Don't wake her up.

In reading this journal, I'm astounded by how much has happened since last year. Since I lost my job at the oil company—the TEC, the job-hunting, the bouts with vasculitis, diabetes, the hours spent putting ice packs on my ankles, fighting the diabetes with cold drinks, Popsicles, the horrible greasy taste in my mouth.

Putting the house up for sale. Realtor and his wife taking me to their church. Being healed. Not using the cane any more.

Being called back to the bank in Nov. The kids coming in Dec. Taking on new job responsibilities.

I'm feeling okay about myself. Evolving into a competent person, able to tell the trustee "I don't take shorthand" and not dying from it. Or getting fired.

Miracle after miracle.

The house payment being lowered.

The lawsuit just might go this next time.

Oh, ye of little faith! Look at what God has done for you already. Don't be afraid.

5/31/90 Thursday p.m.

Tough week at work.

But just remember where I was at this time last year. I'm so grateful. I was so sick for so long. Physically, emotionally, spiritually.

It was a rough time.

Pain. Incapacitating.

Despair. Debilitating.

Weak of limb and heart.

Spirit-less, or diminished.

Pride is gone

Like my hair.

Slowly coursing down the drain.

How did I survive?

What kept me going

When all common sense whispered:

"Give up. Lie down and die."

Oh, it was so tempting at times!

Never to face the TEC again.

Never to do battle with

The bureaucrats as SSI and Disability

And DHR and TRC and

All the uncaring Alphabet Soup People.
It was indeed humbling
To submit to the demands
Of a mere child Social Worker
Who earned maybe five dollars an hour
Just so I could get my electric bill paid for a month.
"I shouldn't have to be here," I thought.
"I'm a good person. I work hard for what I have."
Yet I'm with the unemployed
Standing in interminable lines
As if we had nothing better to do.
I could be resting. Or looking for a job.
My legs refused to hold me up some days.
But who cares?
Does God really care?
I wonder.
I wonder what lessons I'm learning?
Patience. Humility.
Couldn't I learn that an easier way?
I know how I pulled through.
I prayed.
And God answered.

6/24/90

Lots of growth lately.
Some pain.

I'm thinking of going back to school again. Paralegal? I really enjoyed working with the legal aspects of my job. The lien releases, filing papers, etc. I'm praying about it.

Going to court on 7/23 at 9:30. Got to pray about that—a lot.

I bought a book on lupus—*the writer is full of shit*. She rattles on and on about "the sister moon" and her husband is an s.o.b. and finally, she thinks she is cured of lupus.

Bullshit.

She also asks: "What if I were alone, without family—no one to cater to me?"

She'd have to do as I do: Cope.

I told Nancy I hated to even mention lupus to her. I felt like I was bringing it up too often and she would be/is getting tired of it. She assured me that wasn't the case. I don't want to talk about it all the time.

But I do want to celebrate my little triumphs with her. Like going to Shakespeare in the Park—after cleaning house all day and going to a meeting. This time last year, it was impossible to do almost anything.

I noticed the sky at sunset, the stars above the stage at the park last night—and thought: "I may never see this again. It is so beautiful, I'll miss it so."

But where I will be will be even more beautiful, I believe. I will be sad to leave, but no "thing" lives forever. And nothing lasts forever. Not a life. Not a sunset. Not a sunrise. It all changes. Life into death. Sunlight to darkness.

There are days when life is just too complicated. I think sometimes it might be easier if I could just go to the mountains and live in a tent. Drink water and eat berries and wait out my days without the hassle of job, bureaucracies, regulations, bills, and cars needing inspections, for God's sake. A dammed imposition on my time and energy.

Just leave me alone, all you people in control of my life: IRS, SSI, Social Security, DHS, the bank—everyone who wants another piece of me.

You can't have any more of me. My spirit, by God, is mine and mine to keep.

7/8/90

When I related to my friend Nathan how I had negotiated for benefits, he didn't act surprised, or pleased, even. As though he expected me to have done that. At first, I felt slighted. I felt like he should have said, "Atta girl" but it's like he expected it of me to have enough guts to do it. He's not my therapist, anyway. I was just reporting to him, not looking for his approval. Don't need it.

I did at one time. But that was before I started getting well.

Lupus is still in abeyance. Funny how I can put it in its perspective now. It doesn't dominate my life as it used to. It's a large part of it, but not all.

102

7/15/90 Sunday a.m.

Dream. I have been on a mountaintop. A vista with a botanic garden building. I took off my pearls (I am with 2 women) and lay them on the grass. We go down the hill for a while, then I ask them if they saw my pearls. One asks the other and she says, "Yes," but somehow I have to go get them myself. They go with me.

I wake up.

7/22/90 Sunday

Can't stand it any longer. Evading the issue. The issue is my fear about going to court tomorrow. Again.

I told Nancy that I dreaded most of all the possibility of not just me "losing," but Doug "winning." Again. As he always has. Will take my crucifix with me.

Maybe the dream meant: "Casting pearls before swine?"

Trust God, once again.

8/4/90 Saturday a.m.

I told Nancy I thought God was jerking me around. It has taken me this long to write about the court date. Doug has paid for a jury. One more time, I get to wait. My lawyer said it's not a jury matter, and I agree.

I was in shock.

I made an appt. with my atty. Sherman King to ask questions. Yes, he said, he didn't want to go to trial, but only because it was nonsense. He does that all the time. He said he would file a Motion for Summary Judgment, first. I told him I was going to CA and he said let them work around our schedule for a change.

I was able to (a) feel the anger and (b) ask questions.

Also, on the job interviews:

The legal dept. fiasco. I had the appt. right after my court "no show"…well, at 2 p.m., it went that badly. I felt I was being chastised for having had 8 jobs in 8 years. (Little did he know there were more than that!)

I shot right back "yes"—which one in particular did you want to know about? (Who said that?)

I also heard my prospective employer say that mistakes were sudden death.

I thought, *"You son of a bitch. You just lost me."* This job was not for me, I knew. In my gut. I listened to it.

I learned to ask questions. And trust my instincts.

My biggest problem today is a broken dishwasher.

9/9/90

Back from CA last week. Tired. We had a good time. I probably shouldn't have gone to the beach as I now have a rash all over my neck, chest, arms and thighs. I sat under an umbrella and covered up—but that wasn't enough.

Have a drs. appt. tomorrow. Will see how I've done off the Imuran.

Sick today. Sick yesterday. Sinus problems. And the rash is really bad. We'll find out tomorrow. I paid bills, cleaned house…. Did a lot despite being sick.

10/14/90 Sunday

I Begin Stephen Ministry….

Lots going on. I told the trustee last week—"Maybe it's good for you to finish this up quickly, but I'm not feeling too good about it. I have to find something else."

I was surprised to hear myself say that. He said, "Don't worry. You're going to be taken care of."

I said, "Well, I know the others were going to get a severance package and I wondered if I was included."

He said, "You will be amply compensated."

I don't know what he meant by that, but I have a feeling it's good. More than I could ask for, maybe.

Also, they paid my 3 mon Sanus bill. No questions asked. It still might work out with some people who were still in the bank building who needed help.

Health is good. Dr. Morton said the Prednisone could cause my weight gain. Now, he tells me!

Been walking every morning at 5:30. Put on the radio station and hear a Bible study. Several years ago, I would have made fun of listening to a Christian radio station. Some of it is a bit much, I think. Too fundamentalist for me. But I choose what I like.

1/1/91

Happy New Year! "Cascading multiple thoughts."
I'm old. I'm fat. I'm unattractive.
These are feelings.

These are real feelings. I try to remember that what's on the inside counts, and then, everybody looks at the outsides.

Got to wear my snazzy new black suit to see Van Cliburn last night. New hairdo and perfect makeup. Yet I felt "less than" when in the pressure of all the "money talks"

God, relieve me of the bondage of self. God has been so good to me. I had gas in my car—it ran—I got food for my body and my soul—my bills are paid—I have a job (today) I have friends and family—the sun is shining…Well, all things considered, I'm doing okay this 1-1-91.

3/20/91 Wednesday 7 a.m.

Been too busy to write. Avoiding it. Might learn something. Feeling somewhat "down" today.

I know I'm grieving for the old job. Not a new one in sight. Temp work is keeping me afloat. Dysfunctional bunch I worked with last week.

Stressed out, job-wise. Temp work can be the pits. Interviewed for 2 jobs Thursday.

Sanctuary

In church today I felt again
That I lived before...in the church.
The church of long ago
When candles flickered in the nave
And footsteps echoed on stone.

3/20/91 7 a.m.

I dreamed of cars driving into a tunnel. They were jammed in the tunnel and couldn't come out. I asked the person next to me (God?) what was happening and how could this log jam break. He said, "Everybody, be very quiet." And we were and the cars came out. Wow!

Be still and know I am God?

Need to replenish myself—renew—sad. I feel sad. For everyone and everything.

4/91

How did I feel as a child moving from pillar to post, never staying long enough in one place to put down roots, like the flowers my mother never planted, because, as she said sadly, she wouldn't be there to watch them bloom?

I suppose no one ever saw me "bloom," either. I always *came* that way—complete, to their eyes. And I left before they ever had a chance to see me flourish.

I was always, always, cheerful, obedient, kind, clean, studious and "pleasant." I never talked back, I did as I was told, and I didn't rock anybody's boat. If I ever disagreed with anyone, I couldn't say so—I just pretended it didn't matter and just walked away, or brightly changed the subject. This was my public face.

At home, in private, I was much the same, but add lonely and quiet. I spent my time daydreaming, when I wasn't studying or doing homework, or reading or writing. I loved to read, to listen to music, on the AFN radio, with its "You are There" program. Once such captured my imagination that, a year or so later, in the 9th grade, I did a full-blown research paper on Pompeii, which, as we all know, was covered with ash after the eruption of Mt. Vesuvius in 79 A.D. There!

At 8 or 9, I played with a homemade dollhouse that I loved, because it was made by me. It was an overturned, on-its-side orange crate. I made cardboard furniture and placed it carefully in the rooms. I cut window curtains from the Sears Roebuck catalogue (much to my mother's dismay) and used the cloth samples as rugs for the floors. My dollhouse had a swimming pool (a pocket mirror) in the back yard. It had a white picket fence (pipe cleaners) around it. I peopled it with paper dolls drawn by my mother and/or cut from magazines.

So my fantasy life was rich.

I had friends, too, of course. My best friend in the 8th grade was Janie Elmore—the general's daughter. My parents encouraged that. But I think of the subtle ways they discouraged me from associating with a CWO's daughter—Sybil Watson was, incidentally, a hell of a lot more worldly than Janie, who was so sheltered.

Sybil was the one who told me about condoms.

She was only partially right, but then, I didn't know that at the time.

So my friendships were limited by my status as an officer's daughter. Nor could I date an enlisted man.

My hurts came most often when I had to leave one place for another. I couldn't cry. I was told not to. That I would make new friends in the new place.

You would think that my worst hurt would have been when my father would leave. As in 1946—3rd grade. He was just gone one day. To the Far East. Mother cried then, when we found out where we were to go. She must have been scared to death. But she never told me. She held it all in. Like a "good soldier."

So I did, too. Our passport picture shows two females and one little boy with "dead eyes." Pain obscures any other emotion.

I just hated going to school in a new place. What would they think of me? Would I fit in? I always did, of course. I ingratiated myself into the leaders' pack. The best. The most. It was too dangerous to choose any other crowd.

I practiced my smiles. Girl Scout? Solemn? Peter Pan collar? To show up year after year, in new school after new school was truly terrifying. It's a good thing I didn't know it. For I put on my best smile, the bravest front I knew, and went in.

I excelled in school, of course. Math was the exception. I missed a lot of math. Decimals defeated me. Fractions weren't fun. But English and history were great. When I heard that Alexander the Great wept because he had no more worlds to conquer, I wept, too. I think I knew how he felt.

To this day, I cannot claim a home. When someone asks, where are you from, I take a deep breath and begin, "I was an Army brat…"

"Oh, that must have been so interesting," they exclaim.

Actually, I want to yell, I wish I had gone to one school in one town and had friends from kindergarten. That I graduated from high school with, for God's sake, who held my hand when I cried over grades, a boyfriend, one of my best friends betrayed me…Which they never did because they never had a chance to—first of all because I was always so damn good, that if she wanted my boyfriend, I would sort of capitulate and pretend I didn't want him anyway, and second, mostly because I wasn't ever in one place long enough to accomplish making best friends, boyfriends, or enemies.

My childhood was not normal. I grew up too fast. I was not familiar with my emotions. I was a companion to my mother at an age when most mothers and daughters are not speaking to each other. Although I had two younger brothers, I was essentially an only child. I was six years older than my kid brother, and I'm not well acquainted with him now. My baby brother was born when I was 14 and I was his surrogate mother.

5/4/91 Saturday

Storming. Winds and rain lashing at the house. Mayfest is on the agenda. It's 4:20 and we're supposed to leave at 6:00. No way. Too bad since I wanted to hear the symphony.

Tomorrow (Sun) I get commissioned as a Stephen Minister. Should be the start of an interesting time of my life. My life—yes. I am paying attention to it now.

I finally got to court.

I arrived at court early (of course) and then Doug came and he tried to make conversation.

He retreated to the opposite side of the room.

Our lawyers arrived and went into counsel with the master of the court. I opened my prayer book and Doug filled out magazine subscriptions, I think. (I heard him tearing out perforated cards, anyway.) He then paced the halls. My prayer book and my crucifix comfort me in my hand.

My lawyer came out and said, *"The master of the court is telling Doug he's full of shit. How much does he owe you?"*

I was glad I had calculated it prior to going into court—*"$9300,"* I said. Two years, plus Oct. and May of one year—1988 and 1989. He returned to the conference.

Finally, we were called to the bench.

The judge looked sternly at Doug—I was shaking—and pointed to a copy of the divorce decree.

"It says here," he began, and I knew I had won.

"And it says here," he continued, referring to the passages applying to the 121 months contractual alimony, and the "assumes all debts as of May 6, 1982."

"He owed, he didn't pay, and he must." Was the gist of it. Judgment granted. No jury trial.

He has the right to appeal. And probably will.

Stressed out as I was, I added to it by going to two interviews at yet another oil company. The first was awful sounding. Second might be okay.

God, help me find the job I'm supposed to have. I couldn't stand it Friday. I asked for another assignment.

5/4/91 Saturday 10 p.m.

It doesn't take much to make me happy. Just got back from Mayfest where we heard the symphony play the 1812 Overture—America the Beautiful and Stars and Stripes Forever...all complete with fireworks and cannon fire in appropriate places. Loved it. It was a cool evening. Perfect.

> 1812 Overture, complete with cannon
> In appropriate places
> Thrills the crowd.
> But I enjoy the church bells
> As I did in Europe.
> In many ways, Europe is
> More civilized than we are...
> Church bells pealing are much more—
> Subtle, than waking to a buzzing clock.
> So I enjoy the Overture
> With its timpani
> And cannon burst
> And smile to myself as I hear the bells
> The sweet, gentle church bells
> In the midst of a war.

5/7/91 Tuesday

Still stressed out. Tired of being tired.
Is there anything more to life than work, go home, go to bed?
I hate my job.
I feel cheated, somehow.
After having a great job, now must I regress?
Not enough money, ever.
I feel like running away—
Sell everything and move to CA
Start all over.

Am I being unreasonable?
I don't know.
It is an option, after all.
Cat wants affection.
I yell at her. Poor cat.
What am I afraid of?
Growing old—alone.
Growing old—poor
Growing old—dying.

5/11/91 Saturday 3 p.m.

Another damn same old Saturday. Tired. Got up and went to the lab for more blood tests this a.m. First thing. No coffee. Came back, showered, etc., and met the Lunch Bunch for brunch at Harrigan's.

My friend Nathan was correct. I am a hedonist. I like my comforts and fun. Want to go and do—preferably with someone, but can't...no energy—tired most of the time; no money—damn! No one to do it with—double damn!

7/10/91 10:30 p.m.

Went to see counselor, KW, today. I was feeling fragmented. Too busy/too slothful all the time. Described how *"the black cloud descended on me" when I come home every night.* I either run or do nothing...no balance.

She listened, asked about my family of origin (of course) (Family in Oregon, ha, ha) and made some suggestions:

Keep a journal. I had to confess I do and she emphasized that I do it every night. Good, bad, or indifferent.

Write my biography, and cry. Well, God knows I have plenty to cry about. Where to start? "I am born..."

Don't know what I'm depressed over. She surmises I've been depressed since I was very young. This is where the writing

111

comes in. And looking at old pictures. What was going on with me then? And my parents, brothers, etc.

Write. I also told her about my writing and how I love it, but haven't done it, lately.

Cried a bit. Don't know why except I felt sad. Lost dreams. Lost health. Lost child? Do I feel like a lost child?

Then on to lupus support group.

Found out from discussion *nobody* knows when they've done too much until it's too late. They "hit the wall" too. Good to know that.

Find out how to keep my hats from blowing off, too. Velcro on the inside of the band makes the hat smaller, actually.

8/11/91

Mud Pies

When I was a little girl
I made Mud Pies
Making Mud Pies
Gave me pleasure.
The mud squished through my hands
And I tapped it down
Into the pan,
Satisfied.
Where is that childhood innocence now?
When did I become
"Serious" about life?
When did I lose that joy
Of creating something
Out of nothing?
I can see myself
Even now.
A pig-tailed
Little girl,

Intent on the task of
Mixing water and earth
Into the right consistency
To make
Mud Pies.
The smell of the earth—
The graininess
Of the black goo—
I can still feel it.
Lost, I was,
In my task.
The day was long and sunny.
There was no other goal
In mind
But to make
Mud Pies.
And when I was finished,
I dumped them out
And started
All over again.

8/19/91

God, I'm tired of this lupus stuff.
I'm tired of the medicines
And the lab work
And the doctors' visits.
I'm not equipped for the expense,
You know I could use my money elsewhere.
I'm grateful, understand, that
You have provided for all this—
Insurance that pays most of the expenses,
Transportation to and from the lab,
A doctor that keeps me out of the hospital
And a special group of friends who care.
But oh, God, I get tired of this lupus stuff.

Amazed I haven't written in this journal since August. A lot has happened. New job. Feeling better. Losing weight. Woody and Terri will both be here for Christmas.

Load has lightened. Taking antidepressants at night. Sleeping better.

Ten inches of rain last week. I would have felt so depressed, but even with the time change, I'm okay. Tired after a full day's work, but who isn't?

Cold. Chance of snow. This early. We didn't have an autumn. God, I love autumn. That bittersweet time of year. Warm, sunny days, cool nights, went straight from hot days to rain for a week and then, cold. I feel cheated, somehow, I guess for the autumn I should have had.

Norther

Cold wind rattles the shutters.
Wind chimes no longer gently sing
Soft lullabies, but hard rock.
Heater hums, electric blanket goes on my bed.
Coats emerge from the closet, and
Hats, and where are my gloves?
November, Thanksgiving approaches,
Then Christmas.
I am not ready.
Too much to do.
Not enough money to do it with.
Stress sneaks up in the cold night air
And I long for the autumn that we missed.
The autumn of warm, sunny days
And cool, still nights.
The storybook kind
That you remember better

114

Than it really was.
At least the rains are gone.
Cat curls comfortably on the couch.
She doesn't worry about anything at all.
She knows she'll be fed
And loved and nurtured.
Maybe I should heed my cat's lessons.

11/3/91

In church today I felt again
That I lived before...in the church.
The church of long ago
When candles flickered in the nave
And footsteps echoed on stone.
The choir chanted, deep resonant
Tones followed by boyish sopranos
Lifting their voices to God.
I am a supplicant, kneeling in reverence—
Possibly a nun.
I dwell on the mysteries of God
Even as I genuflect, then kneel
I cannot stop the feeling of having
Been there before in another time
In another life
I do not believe this is contrary
To God's law.
I believe He has gifted me
With a look into my past
So I may treasure the present
Even more.
Peace. Reverence. The priest
Imparts the blessing of God Almighty,
As He did once, long ago.
I am changed.
But the church is the same.

7/1/92

Couldn't find "my book" tonight. Chaos reigns in my house. I am moving. Boxes, boxes. Junk. Garage sale items. Decisions. So I decided to just make a new journal.

7/25/92 Saturday 10:30 p.m.

Moved, at last. Been here one week in my new apt. Love it. Quiet, tree-shaded, everything fits. Wind chimes are up. I sat here this afternoon and listened to the wind chimes singing softly. The wind rustled through the trees. Thank you, God, I thought, as I rocked gently in the rocker.

Feeling a bit guilty about having to let the house go. But, I reminded myself, I had no choice.

It's the economy.

I'm not the only one this is happening to.

I'm not a bad person.

I tried my best.

I offered partial payments.

I tried to pay the full payment, but I need to eat and put gas in my car. Reason prevailed. My air conditioner would "blow" any minute. As I left the house last week, Karen, next door, was waiting for the a/c repairman. Thank you, God, I thought as I drove away.

Bob put the ceiling fan up in my bedroom. Yea! Tomorrow will do the other stuff. I'm making a pot roast. Clydie will come over, as her a/c is out. One more "proof" that I'm doing the right thing.

Grateful for: My friends. My family. My new apt. My new life. Freeing. The sun coming up in my bedroom window.

8/9/92

Bone-Dead Tired

I dislike fatigue.
Hate it, in fact.
It makes me think I'm dying.
Which I am, by degrees.
Lupus won't leave me alone.
It sneaks up on me to
Bite me in the ass.
Just a nip, here and there.
A warning—a threat—a presence.
I can't do what I did before.
Damn it to hell!
Insidious infirmity!
Bad enough to be old (-er)
And alone—
Without this—this intruder.
I struggle to church.
I am comforted, for a time.
I want to go and do after.
But my body rebels
"Take me home," it pleads.
Even as I chirp to my friends
"I'm fine."
I'm not fine.
I'm dying. By degrees.
Damn!
I want to live before I die.
Travel. Laugh—love.
Read. Write. Talk to my family.
I don't want a trip to the cleaners
To be a major ordeal.
The climb up the stairs—
Just breathing, sometimes

117

Is more than I can bear.
If I had run a marathon—
Or worked all day in a field
Picking cotton, or plowing, or gardening—
I could understand this fatigue.
But I have done ordinary things—
But I have an un-ordinary disease.
I keep forgetting about "That."
Better respect me, it whispers.
Slow down. Rest. Forego the temptations
To run, and play and talk to friends.
Rest, recoup. Remember—
You have lupus.
Lupus laughs. And waits.
Who will win?
I will. Today.
Today I choose to listen.
Another day, Lupus!

11/17/92

I just read what I wrote way back in Sept.
You'd think that things (and I) would have changed.
NOT! I still feel:
Less than, shame, fearful, deprived, restless, irritable and discontent, lonely, definitely so, at this time, resentful, jealous of others' possession, talents, and praise.

I'm tired of these feelings.

I'm tired of being poor—or of feeling poor. Not managing well? I need—God, you know I need to be able to make my bills (on time) and still have enough left over for medical emergencies, car repairs and a movie out, every so often, without feeling fearful.

I'm a child who is lost. Put me on the path, I pray. Increase my faith. Relieve me of my disbelief. Keep me from waking in fear at 3 a.m., trembling inside from the devil's taunting: "*You're*

118

going to be a bag lady. You'll lose this apartment, just like you lost your house. You can't do anything right. You'll never succeed at taking care of yourself. You need a man to do that, but since you can't choose one wisely, why bother? Just get on with it, stupid woman. Just give up. Life is tough. You can't make it. Might as well lie down and die, right now. Don't be a burden to your kids. Your parents won't have to worry about you any more, either."

God, I hate those thoughts. I know they are lies of the devil.

I need a sign, dear Lord. A visible, clear, certain sign that you are with me. That I don't have to continue feeling this way...that the devil will no longer come to my side during the dark hours when I am weakest.

Lupus and Me

My enemy, my companion
This chronic disease has moved in
And set up housekeeping
In my body
Without my permission.
Most days, we co-exist,
This gypsy and me.
I tolerate her— "Lupe"—
Up to a point.
She tolerates me—
Up to a point.
It hasn't come easy.
In the early days of her encampment,
Nobody knew what "It" was.
What caused my joints to radiate heat?
To ache, day and night—
Despite all the medicines
Fired at her.
We didn't know where she would strike next.
Where she would get the chutzpa.

I co-exist with a chronic illness.
I tolerate its presence—to a point
It tolerates me—to a point.
When first diagnosed,
It had the upper hand.
And wrists and knees and ankles.
Pain was my companion,
My enemy.
My burden.
For a long, long time,
Nobody knew what "It" was.
My Frustration increased
In direct proportion to my doctors' visits.
"I don't know," two or three admitted, glumly.
As if I had defied all their premises.
"Rheumatoid arthritis," one physician
Intoned solemnly.
"Look at those beautiful, swollen knees,"
She said almost gleefully.
If I had had the strength,
I would have taken a swing
At her jaw.
As it was, all I could manage was
A slow protest:
"No, I don't think it's rheumatoid arthritis."
She, the physician, looked at me,
The patient,
As if I didn't know
What my body was feeling.
The diagnosis just didn't fit.

I'm Going Back to School, at My Age!

One success, however, came about by my asking The Texas Rehabilitation Commission for help—and I am returning to school, after 3 years—so far, full-time—for two years at TCJC, with TRC paying books and tuition and a small expense check every week. I am in the Mental Health Program and my goal is to finish at TCJC with my AAS, work part-time in the MH field and continue at UT Southwestern Medical School in Dallas, for my BA in Rehabilitation Science.

Working with people in chronic pain.

1/16/93 Saturday

Xmas Is Over, Kids Gone
No Job
Fired, Again

Feeling betrayed.

Angry, hurt. Why?

And he's trying to avoid unemployment comp. I had to deal with the TEC over this yesterday. Went into a real tailspin. No good. But I stopped it quick.

There are more horses' asses than there are horses.

Therefore:

I can't beat myself up for once again going through this. Some things can't be avoided.

I've avoided dating jerks.

I need to work, and sometimes I don't recognize the jerks before I work for them.

Sometimes, it's THEM.

Positives:

My car is paid for.

My rent and bills are current.

I'm working temporary for two weeks—maybe $3-400).

The temp company had an assignment for me...will probably come up with some more. If not, I'll sign with another.

I passed my typing test at City Hall. Carmen, bless her, told me. I got my notice to call for an interview time.

All who know me tell me that he was wrong to let me go.

When I get a new job—or if I can just draw unemployment for a while, it will be good for me to reflect and grow and maybe write!

2/10/93

Feeling alone. Job-hunting still on going. Temp work at Hampton-Azle a learning experience.

Still having difficulty with resentment and fear. Found myself "wiped out" and on the couch last Sat. night and started crying over a TV show...shows from the past. First began weepy eyes—no real feeling at that time...just found myself weeping. Then came feelings. Great sobs...why was I crying?

I couldn't cry then. Crying now over the lost past...up to and including the recent past?

I am fearful that I might get another "real" job and get fired again.

Temp work okay but no benefits.

If I get sick—no pay.

If I work temp—no health ins.

I'm screwed.

2/14/93

Up and Down—Ash Wednesday. Appropriately named.

Today more down than up.

And it rains. Pours down.

And I don't feel like going to Ash Wednesday HE.

And I get a note from the TEC that I must appear and give them a look at my driver's license and SS card, which I had done and because of their mistake in not entering it into their

122

computer, I have to be inconvenienced.

And I'm not any closer to a job.

And I'm achy because of the weather.

And I've temporarily lost my support system because of my work hours.

And I'm still grieving over the job loss and probably over my marriages, crappy as they both were.

And my health problems won't go away. You'd think I'd be reconciled to them by now...I'm not "cured" but "healed" in spirit, at least. Making peace with lupus at least most of the time.

"Surrender" sounds like it.

"Retreat" is probably more what I'm doing.

Resting—gathering strength for the next round of life.

2/26/93

Yesterday was a "demon" day.

Drove to TEC to show them my driver's license and SS card "to register for work"—I had done that the first time I went out, but they said, "It's not in the computer." So I had to do it again.

Came home and called Azle (NW Hampton)—no work today, there. So I went to see about food stamps and Medicaid. Waited from 10:30-11:15. Then was told to come back at 1:00.

Had a good lunch at nearby Luby's. I deserved it.

Went back to DHS—finally got called at 1:30. Bottom line is I "make too much money to qualify." They don't take into consideration medical expenses. So I asked about Medicaid. I need to be either pregnant or over 60. Or have a child living with me.

No dice—no luck. SOL.

Got a voucher for $21 for food, though.

Went to the school district to register as sub secretary.

Stopped by and got my car inspected.

The food voucher must be redeemed on E. Lancaster's Safeway or Jacksboro Highway on certain days at certain times. I said to hell with it and stopped by Albertson's for bread, milk, eggs, etc., for a total of $23. Will use the $21 voucher later for frozen foods, when I can go to E. Jesus in the daylight.

2/26/93 Friday

A thought. Why not work in the Hampton temporary pool and get on their HMO? And get prescripts paid for—or almost—$5 per? Find out how much they'll take out of my checks…will it be worth it. Or, I could go to the county hospital.

3/8/93 Monday

Blue Monday. No work scheduled for today. So I'm "on the street," instantly. In my mind. Negative thoughts flood me. I feel constricted. Tight. Holding my breath. It's not healthy to do that, I know. I find myself almost paralyzed by fear. I remember when I was married to Doug and just sat in the rocker. Afraid to move. No wonder my body rebelled. Constant stress hurt it—damaged it—as if it had been beaten. No wonder I feel as though I've been "beaten up."

I sit beside the window and look at the tree. It's blooming. Bees gather around its blossoms. Birds are building nests. The tree is not concerned about anything. God planted it there and it's just doing what a tree is supposed to do—bloom in the spring, give shade in the summer, shed leaves in the fall, and endure the winter.

My "winter" is gone. It's spring. I'm alive. Perhaps not living an ideal life, but alive, nonetheless.

I've been in worse spots than this, and walked through it. I remember when I was in the hospital. Fired. Looking for a job while carrying a cane and wearing a wig and going home each day crying with pain from my swollen legs…rubbing ice on them. God carried me thorough that time…why do I disbelieve now?

I need to grieve. I need to rage. I need to cry for my soul. I have been wounded in many ways, over many years.

I feel my energy is not being focused, but scattered. What is important? What is necessary? What do I need right now? Rest? Probably. I have drawn on my reserves too often, like an overdrawn bank account. There is not much left to draw from. But I ask: "Is it lupus or is it life?" Is this normal to feel so down—discouraged?

I will get through this.

And come out stronger.

3/9/93

I took such good care of myself today. *I turned down a job assignment.*

Sounds crazy? But—when I got to the SW Rehab Hospital, the HR person told me I needed to take a TB test because I would be "exposed to patients who have TB."

Well, all kinds of bells went off in my head—and I listened! I told her, "I can't do that. I have lupus and have had lung involvement."

Called TEC and left a message re: my check. They called back later and I'm to get 2 checks for a total of $224 mailed yesterday.

And this morning I also called my attorney and left a message on his machine re: address change, phone #, that I had lost my house, my job, I'm getting sick again, *and I need my money.*

Think I've done enough?

I really want to go back to school…

4/11/93

Easter!

He is Risen! He is Risen Indeed!

Wonderful church music this morning. I glory in the music and the ritual.

Tonight I'm watching *The Sound of Music*. And crying. As I always do. Grieving over that part of me that's still a kid who lived there? Am I idealizing my life there?

125

It wasn't perfect…but I felt a deep love of the land, the people, the church bells that rang every day, calling their faithful to worship, morning noon and evening.

Maybe I lived in a fairy-tale world? I was—or I felt safe…yet independent, exploring as I did the city of Linz. Climbing the hill up to the Spanish Guard Tower and lying in the grass, gazing up into the sky. Turning now and again to look down onto the Danube River flowing, like time itself, on and on…towards the great ocean.

Mourning that time—that place…where the future lay before me…all promise. All mine to look forward to.

What happened to me? What happened to that young girl?

Life intruded, I suppose. Reality. How can I get that back? That feeling of—what? Total one-ness? Yet independent—with the world?

Well, I have some of that now. God gave me a place to sit and look out at the trees. Just to BE. Well, I guess I just get to grieve and not try to figure it out.

That crazy woman at H&R Block told me I owed—gasp—$2329 because of the foreclosure

Nancy, telling her my problem: "Do you believe she's right?"

Why, that had never occurred to me.

"Helen at H&R Block" represented Authority to me, and God knows, I don't ask questions of Authority.

So, I decided maybe she was wrong. And also I was reminded that I paid just a bit more than that for my car…my car! I could re-finance my car!

That was a way out.

I felt better, but after the meeting, I couldn't pray the Our Father. Just let tears run down my face. Too choked up to pray.

And Andrea came over to tell me she appreciated what I had said last meeting and what was the matter?

Now, I didn't know her at all. Just met her last meeting. I wouldn't have said anything to her about my taxes, but this time I just blurted it out. Amid sobs, and she grinned and said, "*You don't have to pay that. The foreclosure has nothing to do with your taxes. I'm a CPA. Let me look at it.*"

Well, well. *God laughs again.*

I went right back to Helen and got my stuff back. Told her my folks were coming up and we'd take it to their CPA.

I offered to pay her for her time.

She said, "No," and handed me my package.

As I turned to leave, she said, shaking her finger at me, "But it's the rules!"

4/20/93

Tomorrow is my birthday anniversary. 55! Mom sent a pretty card and a $55 check and words of encouragement.

Spent the morning at JTPA taking evaluations. Everything came out for artistic, creative—counselor, teacher, and *writer...* not a secretary.

I feel validated and affirmed. I'm not surly, or willful, or incompetent, I'm literally not cut out for that kind of work. Too expressive, free, verbal. High verbal skills no surprise.

Also I have changed from INFJ to ENFJ—extrovert. It must mean I'm growing. Able to and more willing to initiate conversations, be more responsive, etc. Better at communicating —need to practice on conflict.

I am sitting by the window, not thinking of much, when a thought, or feeling comes over me: "My problems with my father are being resolved." It felt so good...so true...so peaceful. And then my friend.... Dad calls to tell me he's building me a computer, and putting Word Perfect 5.1 on it. Wow!

What I'm trying to say is: I'm so content now. Finding "my right living"—being myself.

Tomorrow I deal with SS re: disability. Just in case I need it.

Terri sent me a framed picture of herself and Woody.

Even though I dislike being a secretary, I'm still darn good at it, no matter what other bosses said.

127

4/21/93

Temp Work in the Federal Building for the National Weather Service
I Begin Teaching ESL

Birthday! Time for reflection.... Did some deep thinking over the Branch Dravidian thing tonight. The children! But I believe if they had been abused, they may be better off. At least they know God loves them and they won't suffer any more at the hands of their parents, or that crazed David Koresh.

I had a hard time explaining why this person is not really a Christian to these Buddhists! (ESL) Really puts my faith to the test. And I believe even more in my own church's teachings.

4/29/93

Took off this week—got sick on Tuesday—dizziness and ears hurting. Clydie took me to the dr. I have spent entirely too much at the dr. this month.

I think this part-time job will be just fine. That will get the TEC off my back. I can still count on my measly $224 per week. It's keeping me afloat.

God is teaching me something. Maybe it's that I can have this time to write. If I work between 10-2, that leaves the rest of the day to write. At least thru August. Then maybe school. But what to take? I'm open to any suggestions.

5/1/93 Saturday p.m.

Starting to work at TCOM Monday a.m. and helping after 2 p.m. in another area for 5 weeks.

So I'll have just about a full day, each day.

Money situation is just fine. I have what I need today. And then some left over.

5/17/93

No air conditioning. Started going down yesterday afternoon. But I'm not crazy over it. TV just flipped out, too. That, I don't like at all. The a/c is not my a/c to fix...the TV is.

Grieving over my job situation—again.

Talked to Clara at meeting Saturday. She asked me if I knew about the Masters Program: Over 55. I'll also see if Texas Rehabilitation Commission can do something for me.

5/18/93

Okay, God. I need:

A job where I can stay home when I'm sick.

A job I really enjoy and would do for free—like teaching ESL.

Benefits, if at all possible—i.e., sick pay.

And this is why I need the above:

I am, as you know, 55 yrs. of age. Nobody will hire me as a secretary—with benefits.

Besides that, my resume looks awful. Too many jobs and gaps.

My health is definitely a factor. Stress is making me ill. Today I had spastic colon—why? Too much stress at work.

Well, God, thank you very much. I'm really scared, you know.

I look in the mirror and see a middle-aged, frumpy old gal. Please help me lose some weight. I know it's not good for me. Besides, it makes me look old and frumpy.

Tomorrow I go to JTPA for this workshop. I don't want to go. It's a waste of time. I want them to tell me now what I should be doing.

I don't think secretary/medical transcriptionist is it. Or is it? I could do that at home.

5/21/93

I'm so tired. Lonely. Angry, too. I want to go out on Friday nights, like everybody else. To a movie—or somewhere. But I'm so tired.

I must remember, I have lupus. Lupus makes you tired. I'm also 55. My body is tired from that age, too.

I have much stress in my life lately. No job. Don't want to keep doing the same thing over and over: Get a job, any job, lose it, go on unemployment, get a job, any job, lose it…Nuts to that. I have a chance now to do what I really want to do…counsel others, and/or write/prepare resumes—teach ESL/do medical transcriptions. Lots to do before next week.

6/1/93

My friend Nancy's husband Bryan died today at 6:30 a.m. We knew the angels were gathering weeks before. We could feel their presence.

I had a resentment that I had to go ahead and keep my appt. with Clara at the TRC. Would rather have stayed at Nancy's. But Clara encouraged me to get my MHMR degree—AAS & CAADAC. I had to go to NW campus to get my transcript evaluated and then to NE campus for the "real" evaluation for the MHMR program. And I still have to call the supervisor of that dept. (Dean? Do they call them "deans" at TCJC?)

Anyway, I didn't get out of there until 6:30 and came home and called to tell them I couldn't come tonight for the ESL class. There just isn't enough of me to go around today.

Clara also pointed out that medical transcription is probably the most stressful job around. I had to agree. MHMR is the thing I want to do and she says I can do it. No sweat. Possibly intern at an agency to get more CEUs.

Mind is a jumble. Very tired.

7/8/93

How's My Schoolgirl? My Father Asks

Wow. Had appt. w/Clara at TRC this afternoon. *I'm going to school!* What's more, I'll get $25 per week for summer and then $50 per week in the fall/winter.

I told Clara that was my medicines. Now I can pay for them. (Instead of going 2-3 times a month and getting only enough for 1 week.)

I can hardly believe it.

School. Going to have a career change. No more secretarial shit work. It will no doubt be *another kind of shit work*, but it won't be like the shit I had: Working to make somebody else rich, while I got dumped on.

So excited. But not so excited over my tests. I'm a perfectionist, fearful of criticism, didn't do well in math (I'm surprised it's 7th grade—would have thought it was just 3rd grade). I'm also determined and persistent. I have all the traits necessary to go to school.

I also was diagnosed as having an "adjustment disorder" due to lupus, with signs of recent abuse in marriage. No shit.

Much work ahead of me.

7/20/93 Tuesday

And I'm Back on a School Campus

One week of school under my belt. Will have a test next Thursday. Still need to do a lot of reading.

Went to Boerne this weekend. Dad was installed as Worshipful Master of the Masonic Lodge—he and Mom are held in high esteem, as evidenced by the large turnout. Good to know that.

131

8/13/93

What a difference 2 weeks can make. I'm going to CA and OR to see my kids. Thanks to the "Trip Fairy" (Liz and Don). Now I all I need is a bit of cash for all those little things…a Coke on the plane, tips for the porters, etc.

Well, lots of stuff going on. School is over. Get my grades Tues. A or B. It's okay to get a "B."

Also got news today from the CPA—looks like I'm off the hook with the IRS. I get back $236, but I owe her $200—"Good news, bad news." At least I'm out of that fear now.

9/4/93

Miracles—My Life Has Been Full of Miracles

School—through the program.
Trip to see my kids.
My "God car."
My brother, family around.
My health changes for the better.
Mental health okay—better.
Trip to Terri's…left Tuesday p.m. and arrived at Orange Co a bit late. But Terri is a bit late, too. We had a storm over AZ. I was in terror. Spilled Coke all over myself. Oh, well, I survived.

Wednesday

We went and had our pedicures. Had lunch at Taco Poco…served by a real airhead. At Laguna, I think. Had dinner with Terri and friend Darlene at Italian restaurant at the outdoor mall.

Thursday met Jayne for lunch at the Cheesecake Factory. Had lox and bagels. Yum. Then to the island and beach for pix and

132

then that night to Fashion Island for Jazz festival. Fun crowd. Tossed beach ball into crowd. Some of Terri's crowd on cell phones—how California!

Friday spent quietly by the pool—in shelter—till time to leave for Woody's.

Took commuter flight to LA—a small 10-seater plane. Flew at treetop level. No a/c. Mercifully, it's a smooth 20 minutes.

At LAX—I take Delta flight to Portland. It's a 2 1/2 hr. flight. Get to Portland just in time for another commuter flight to Redmond. This is a 30-seater propjet. I'm disappointed, it's dark and I can't see the Cascades. Woody meets me at Redmond. Collect Suitcase from Hell and go to Bend.

Typical bachelor apt. Needs a woman's touch, but it's clean. To bed by 11 p.m. Up around 8:00 and after getting ready—go to breakfast. Then to outdoor museum. Then to a funeral home, where Woody is associated. I'm amazed at him. Then I eat Chinese food—meet some of his friends and then went to see *The Fugitive*. $5 for evening movie. Next day, head home.

School started Monday. What have I done?

First class was Life Span Growth and Development. Not too bad. Then Behavior Mod. Tues. Abnormal Psy. In a.m. 3:30 water aerobics. Then Laws and Standards. Pooped by Friday. No classes Friday.

Laws and Standards will be a bitch. Tough woman attorney. Oh, well. Do the best I can.

9/20/93 Monday

I thought school would be snatched away from me...like a kid. I got my caboose in front of my engine, when the TEC told me my benefits were exhausted.

I bawled and squalled and snot came out of my nose, in the library. I hyperventilated and sobbed all that day and took an exam that night.

I feel so afraid. I feel—value-less. I feel betrayed. I have grief over this dream not materializing.

I feel "less than." Others seem to get what they want, with little or no effort. Certainly not with the obstacles that block my way.

Do I not take the right actions? Is it something I did or didn't do? Why does it seem such a damn struggle just to take care of myself?

Okay, I'll work—at what?

I'm stressed out. School? What about school? Can I manage both? Can I earn enough by temporary work to meet my Oct. rent? Not to mention my bills—electric, car ins. Phone. The basics.

I feel like I've been hung out to dry and I'm twisting in the wind.

I feel almost suicidal. What's the use?

10/6/93

The upshot is that I've re-applied for a grant, resubmitted my claim and it looks like everything's going to work out. Terri paid my rent.

My folks beeped in while I was talking to Nancy and I told them about "no school, no money, and no hope."

TEC called and wants a damn dr's note. Can't they just do things my way? Hell, no. I've got to do things their way. Deal with imperfect people in an imperfect world.

But will get a note tomorrow to take to them. Remember, I live in an imperfect world!

And I'm not perfect, either.

10/19/93

There is a God. Got my TEC checks last week. 3 of them. Went to Dallas for the lupus seminar on Saturday.

It's raining hard. Body achy. Worried about the drive to school.

Need to pat myself on the back for being an adult. When I

went to the TEC with proof of my employment dates—not the 15th of June but the 26th as last day, I had kept a pay stub and showed it to them.

Also Dr. Morton's letter. It just stated I have lupus. But they took it anyway. I acted like I was so surprised that he didn't put the 15th date. "Oh, my—well, I asked for it, but this is what I got."

And just shrugged helplessly and they took it.

Thank you, God. Now I'm working on a grant or a loan.

12/3/93 Friday a.m.

Year in Review

Re-read my journal and wonder how I've survived this year. Miracles, that's how. I wish I had made better progress; you'd think I'd be better by now, but I still doubt God, foolish person that I am.

Rent went up…I can do it…if the TEC will continue to pay. I have to go see them to day and file my claim. Have a seminar this afternoon.

School is almost over. Burned-out folks around me. Made an 80 in Life Span—I know I accidentally missed at least 2, but it would still be a "B" anyway. This is the grade to drop. Turned in 3 papers I worked on all Thanksgiving weekend…Ab. Psy (about panic disorder); B. Mod about my biofeedback for lupus; Laws and Standards about the Mental Health code as applied to the movie *Frances*.

Sometimes I worry that I'm really losing my mind. Maybe I'm just getting older—not old, but just old-er. Sometimes I wonder if this is all worth it—going to school.

Frantically trying to make my rent and bills. But so is everybody else. A girl in water aerobics is considering moving in with her mother since the TEC quit paying her. I urged her to go there and fight for it. Refile her claim.

135

Maybe what I've learned is helping others? Maybe that's the point?

"Cascading multiple thoughts." Christmas is fast approaching. Kids will be here soon. Need to register for school again. But first—Finals. So far, so good on my grades.

Lord, I wish "Authority" had no control over me. I need some measure of control in my life. I know all I can control is my emotions/actions. Some things I have no power over, and that galls me. (The TEC is like the military? I didn't like the military always ruling my life, either.) What more lessons do I need to learn?

I have learned how to be poor.

I have learned how to go to school again.

I have learned how to share my feelings with others.

I probably haven't learned yet to Trust. I nearly always feel betrayed by others, in one way or another.

1/20/94 Friday

School started the 18th...felt overwhelmed for a day or so. 4 classes back-to-back. Might not be such a good idea. I'm out before 2 p.m., though, and have only one morning class, T &Th.

Called my lawyer yesterday. Got a non-answer. As they will do. At least I recognized it as such. He said he'd check the middle of next week. I never did get a "date" from him, even when I said, "The TEC gave me 14 days...how long do they have to get back to me?"

Anyway. The TEC still sends claim forms and I send them back. I have no money coming from them. Not since before Christmas. About the 1st of Dec. Thank God I have my student loan, at least for this month. After this, I will have No Income for a while, until I get a grant, or a job. It's really scary to think I have No Money Coming In right now.

Yet, I have all I need today. Faith cannot coexist with fear.

Such a zoo with the JTPA. I was in the *county* funded JTPA—the one on Highway 80 is *city* funded. I need to see if they have a computer data bank for grants and loans.

Why don't people tell us those things? Why didn't the JTPA—county-funded—say, "Try the City JTPA program?" Bozos.

Also called TRC to ask about my checks. "You should get them the 30th or the 7th of Feb." I'm glad I called and asked, anyway.

God, I ask for your help in finding a way to get an income, or get a grant/loan, etc., so I can continue in school. I truly love it and will love my new career. There are other "older" people in the program, too. I don't know where to look or what to do next. How much of this is mine? How far do I go? Am I doing the right thing? I really need your help, God. I'm doing the best I can, in the faith department.

2/3/94 Thursday p.m.

I'm glad I'm keeping this journal. Even though I don't write daily. Some days are not worth writing about. Ordinary things… non-events. No big deals. Just a routine day.

School is okay. I hope I can continue. I'm tired of being in fear about my finances. 90% of the time I can put it out of my mind.

But the 10% that worries me is Strong! It wakes me early. My heart is pounding in fear. How am I going to pay the rent? My car ins. is due. Electric. Not to mention the other bills and gas money. The TRC let me down re: my checks. I have resentment about that.

2/10/94

TRC came through with $150.

There are many ways to earn money other than the traditional "secretary."

God does work in mysterious ways.

Test in communications = 92.

Took test in Alcohol and Drug Survey…probably 95 or so. No school today due to ice. God is good. I didn't have to get out. Was all warm and safe in my apt. with my black cat in my lap. Only a few small stabs of "financial insecurity fear." I can pay my car tags and car ins. And electric bill. Sanus and rent next to worry about, at the end of the month.

Boy, what I could do with $10,000. I lived—or survived—on $12,000 in '93. So I can do it. If I'm real careful. So far, I've been able to go to a movie about once a week, eat out and enjoy a few things.

Learning so much about myself. The dean suggests all of us (her students) have therapy, so we can be better therapists. I really took her at her word and called my church counselor.

3/2/94

Good News/Bad News

Finally went to the county medical district for meds. I pay only $2 each.

Plus 7 hours of waiting.

It was worth it and I won't have to do that again. They can mail my refills.

GOOD NEWS #2: I WON MY APPEAL.

BAD NEWS: I owe my attorney $350. Will have to pay it out.

GOOD NEWS: My kids are so good. Sent money to old mom.

BAD NEWS: Got a letter re: the foreclosure. Not too concerned; they can't get blood out of a turnip.

Went on to school. Made a 94 in Counseling exam.

4/2/94

Haven't written in a while. Forgot to include my "victory" over the TEC.

I had a decision to make as I left TCJC one afternoon a couple of weeks ago. I "felt" an urge to check the TEC one more time re: 6-7 weeks of unemployment.

I had a feeling I was correct. One part of me, the old one, said, "Oh, why do you even want to bother? You know they'll just tell you you're just wasting your time." I could turn right and go home, or turn left for the TEC.

I turned left.

I asked one woman—the same one who had told me a couple of weeks ago that I was "not entitled to any more benefits" —about: "Don't I need to get 6-7 more weeks after I've been notified my benefits are exhausted?"

She frowned. I added, "See, I filed an appeal, and I won my appeal and got $1700. But I got all mixed up on the dates of payment, so what I'm asking is, is there 6-7 weeks left?"

She said, "Only if you were paid before Jan. 30th." I said the date on my first letter was Jan. 15. She looked it up on the computer and sure enough—I was entitled to 7 more weeks.

I filled out the form, they had not included a form with my last check…and I turned them in the next day. Done.

I got $1700. *Thank God I listened to my "new" tapes instead of my old, self-defeating ones.*

It's a good thing I got the money. I owe $800 in taxes…and on top of all that, tooth problems.

One pulled, last Thursday, then a lot of pain after; next a root canal. Then new crowns to replace the temporary ones.

I sent only $100 with my tax return and let them know I can pay it out. I'll have $500 to do my teeth—root canal.

Hurt like crazy for a few days. Now I'm just tired. Exhausted. And scared.

But maybe a lupus patient who has a tooth extracted is affected more than an "average person." It's only been a week.

I need to sit at my computer tonight, but just don't feel like working on my stuff.

Which really worries me. I have 3 exams next week and 3 papers due before the end of the month.

And maybe I shouldn't have signed up for the Overseas Brats convention on Saturday, since I have a seminar and school on Friday afternoon.

The MHMR interviews were postponed one too many times, because of my dental work. One woman flatly left the message on my machine that "it won't be necessary" to reschedule.

Too bad. I guess I didn't need to work there, with their bad attitude.

> I need a job
> But I need to rest.
> I need to rest
> But I need to study.
> I need to study
> But I need to rest.
> I need to rest
> But I need a job.
> Lord, you know my needs.
> I don't know how I can work
> And study
> And go to school
> And rest.
> You do.

4/9/94

Tired again.

Or, still.

Went to Overseas Brats today—all day—in Dallas. Nobody there from Seoul or Linz, at least from my "era." Met a guy who had gone to high school in Seoul, but it was much later than I!

Joined. Got my T-shirt and bumper sticker. I'd sure like to go to Atlanta in Oct. but—no money—need to work…etc.

Right now, I need to rest. I'm so tired. I'll stay home tomorrow. Not go to church. One reason is Bob and Evelyn are bringing Katie for me to baby-sit while they go to brunch at the Worthington.

I'm really worried about how tired I am…still. Feeling this way for—how long? Too long. At least a couple of weeks.

Fatigue
Creeps over me
Like a dark shadow.
Robs me of joy.
Takes away my zest
For life and friends.
Even though I persist
In doing what I want to do—
Until I can no longer do it.
My body craves sleep
And rest—a lot of rest.
My mind insists
"You're not that tired."
(How tired is "that tired"?)
Oh, how I hate feeling
Tired, weak and weary.
I hate it as much as
I hate feeling poor,
Pitiful, and broke.
God, heal me
If it is your will.
If it is your will
If it is in your Grand Scheme
Of Things
For me to be restored to Health
If not completely
Restored to Health,
Could you please just make it
Where I can feel some energy
90% of the time?
And, God, if it is your will,
Restore me to financial security.
I'm asking only for enough to keep me
Above water—and a bit over for fun.

141

I never had a "home town."

A place where I could be from. When others asked me "Where are you from?" I could only take a deep breath and answer: "My father was last stationed at….And before that, we were in…"

And they nodded politely and moved on, puzzled by my reply.

Overseas Brats understand this dilemma: The litany of posts and bases and rotations.

When others talk about living in the same house in the same town and going to the same school all their growing-up years, I think, and sometimes tell them, "I attended nine schools on three continents. And perhaps twice as many houses, or quarters, as some were."

I learned to speak Korean—a few phrases here and there. And "bastardized German" crept into my high school French—much to my chagrin. "Good try, Marilyn," my French teacher sighed. "But this sentence is only half French—the other half is German."

I studied ancient history in the fourth grade in Seoul Dependents School. I knew where the 38th parallel was long before the North Koreans crossed it and plunged us into war. I had my own private Cold War when the Russians cut off our electricity and I was in the middle of my homework. Not to worry—Coleman lanterns kept handy for just such inconvenience lighted my schoolbooks.

I toured monasteries in Austria and steel mills, and castles. And shopped open-air markets where I bargained for flowers and foodstuffs. I rode in splendor on the Orient Express and was only mildly inconvenienced by Russian border guards demanding our official papers.

As the 38th parallel separated N from S Korea, so the Blue Danube kept Russian Zone and American Zone separate in Linz.

On lazy summer afternoons I climbed the hill to the Spanish Guard Tower and gazed across the water and "felt" the Russians staring back at me.

The Cold War turned hot in 1950 when North invaded South Korea. We were in Europe, on leave in Paris, when word of the invasion came to us. Damn Communists prevented us from completing our vacation as we hurried back to our base in Linz. Damn Russians might "start something" in Europe, my father explained as we hurriedly packed.

I had never heard my father swear before.

It was, however, a swearable occasion.

Nothing happened and life went on—Teen Club dances and movies and school. (You see where my priorities were!) While Korea burned and exploded and we worried about our houseboy, Kim.

My father was called back to Korea as a military advisor, after the Korean War. He went back to our old quarters, HQG27 in Camp Sobingo and took snapshots of what was left of our home. Pockmarked, like a teen with severe acne. The stucco walls were standing, though just barely. Mortar shells, here, air strafing there…And my bedroom over there, with boards across the windows. My school—minus its domed roof. No commissary or p.x. Gone.

We had servants. A matter of custom and necessity for us. But others see that as an attempt to "brag" and "put on airs." Hey, it was just a custom—houseboy named Kim Yung Kyu—3 maids—EE Chung Soo, Moon Sung Che and Mrs. Kim (no relationship to Kim).

Herr Lehner in the basement of our house on the hill overlooking the Danube in Linz. Maria with the gold front tooth and the biggest feet I ever saw, a refugee from Rumania. Katie, the 17-year-old maid who lived with her grandmother and brother, the only family she had remaining, in the DP camp some distance from our quarters in Froschberg.

Servants? Yes. It didn't give us airs. In fact, Janie Elmore, the general's daughter, and I pushed her butler into the swimming pool during a weekend house party (her parents were gone). We probably got into the liquor cabinet, too.

My mother is reluctant to reminisce about Korea. Life was not

143

good to her there. Dad was gone on maneuvers and it was damn cold: minus 35 degrees and miserably hot in the summer. And monsoon rains threatened our sanity. Mom drew paper dolls for me. She played bridge. She didn't drink too much, as many of the wives did. One of the women she played bridge with committed suicide one hot summer night.

I can still hear the tolling of the bell—Ama, Mama, in the still night air.

Life in the compound was hard. We had no running water "except when the houseboy picks up the ten gallon cans and runs with them," Mom wrote to her mother. We had no fresh meat, no milk except Avocet cream, watered down. Mom cooked on a wood-burning stove and we had an icebox. Literally, an icebox. Toilet was flushed with a pull chain. Shower was rigged some way. Our first quarters burned to the ground one cold day. I was in front of the fireplace; Dad was reading close by. I saw the tendrils of smoke rising from the hardwood floor. "Daddy, there's smoke coming out of the floor."

We were out of there in a hurry, got new quarters. Thereafter, no one could use the fireplaces. A potbellied stove was brought into each house and it was placed squarely in the middle of the living room, in a sandbox.

Boy, that played hell with the furniture arrangement.

I went to the Newly Diagnosed Lupus meeting at FW Rehab. Every time I go, I must face the truth of my illness…my disease…lupus. I hate it. I want to do so much.

Have an appt. with Morton at 3:45. I always get just a little "squirrelly" about the time I have to go see him. It reminds me of the inevitability of this disease. The permanence of it. And I get angry.

Angry that I have no money, no job, and no significant other, at least, not now.

I guess I'll love someone and he will love me when it's time. When I'm "weller"—spiritually, and when he is ready, too. In the meantime, I'm loved and nurtured by my friends.

School again tomorrow. The last few weeks. I need to do my papers soon. Tuesday afternoon—Thursday afternoon. Both due before the 27th.

My birthday is Thursday. 56 years on this planet. God has a sense of humor.

4/21/94

56 years old today. Wow. Had a pretty good day. One of my classmates brought warm cinnamon muffins for our usual coffee break after class.

At home—flowers delivered. From Terri. Message on my machine from her…and from Woody. Carmen called and sang an off-key happy birthday. Clydie brought me 2 pr. earrings. Nancy gave me a "plant angel." I need it…And coffee/gourmet and note cards. Called me, too, today. Even when she's hurting.

And Lauri called tonight. "Is this your birthday? I've been thinking all day it must be." She's planted a garden…I have "dibs" on tomatoes.

Went to the county clinic yesterday—to the Arthritis Clinic. Saw a "baby" doctor. Told him Dr. Anderson had diagnosed me in '88. He excused himself and pretty soon, here came "Dr. Dan." He examined me, told me to start wearing my wrist splints again at night. I told him my muscles hurt and he told me I need PT—stretching exercises. So I have an appt. next Tues.

Also, my ankles hurt. Probably residue of the vasculitis? Some neurological damage?

Well, it's been a good day. Oh, yes. I got my hair cut, too. To eliminate "hat hair."

4/25/94

Tornadoes all around. Edgecliff reported a funnel on the ground. Hail fell on the roof, carport, size of marbles.

Came home from school. Got on the couch and slept for one solid hour. I turned in my report on the molecular engineering.

I was the only one who wrote a report. Talk about an overachiever!

Then, Sociology class. Turned in my report (5 extra points) on the Holy-Ghost-ers. Took notes like crazy. Then, on to Speech class where I had to give a 5 min. speech on a profession...so I chose writing. I did better than I thought: a 29.5 out of 30.

Then on to Drug and Alcohol Survey, where I turned in my report (5 extra points) on Mescaline.

I talked to the TRC, both Signe and Clara, and it looks like I'll go to work. Temporary, again. Then I can go to school at night. And the TRC would still pay my $300 month subsistence.

I really am scared about this, God. I worry that I might get sick again. If I'm sick, no work...No work, no money. No money, no place to live.

Am I disasterizing?

Storms all around me. Matching my emotions.

5/9/94

Took my final exam in Survey of Alcohol and Drugs. Then drove in blinding rainstorm to drop off my app. at Hampton for the temp pool. Came home and napped.

Mother's Day...All my kids called. Both girls sent cards. I had already given Mom her "plant angel" and sent her a card. Didn't call. It's okay. I don't feel "obligated" since she was just here.

Well, I found some of my classmates from Linz. A miracle. I don't know what this is all about, or why I'm so excited about it. But I'm finding part of my past...my roots from a rootless past.

I'll find out what it all means in June or November...when I go to the reunions. YEA!

5/12/94

Took my final "final" this morning. Feeling a bit sad about it all coming to an end. At least my classmates from this semester. It feels— familiar—leaving my classmates again.

Funny that this Overseas Brats came about—for me, anyway, at this specific time....

146

Years have passed since I was a girl who went to school in Korea and Austria and other places in between. In Korea, in Seoul, I was only in the fourth grade. Nonetheless, I learned, besides the basic 3 Rs, about Alexander the Great, and Mesopotamia and Egypt, and English history, too. We didn't think it unusual to be sitting in a classroom in Asia where the Russians rattled their sabers quite often. Having no electricity by which to do our homework was no excuse…they did that often, you know, the Russians cut off our electricity, just to annoy us.

Coleman lanterns were lighted and generators guaranteed that "the show" would go on, at the base movie theatre.

My teacher was Mrs. Weed. I can see in my memory my schoolroom—a large room on the ground floor of a huge, old stone building, which reminded me of our own capitol building. At least, to a 9-year-old, it looked that large.

I walked to school in the compound called Camp Sobingo. The p.x. and commissary and hospital were close by. The Red Cross Building was across from the compound gates.

One night, the school auditorium burned. I watched the flames from my bedroom window, and then moved to the kitchen window, where Dad stood. Maybe we won't have school now, I thought. That made me feel sad, somehow, because I liked school. And sure enough, we continued having school. All that burned was the auditorium, which was used as a church and I remember the Hymnals burned.

Earthquakes were common. They woke me but I went back to sleep quickly. No harm done.

The Officers Club and the radio and books and records occupied our time.

I remember Chuckie Sullivan and Billy Gunkel and Jimmy Gunkel. Their parents were Madge and Bill Gunkel. I didn't like their father.

We had no running water. Kim poured water from 10-gallon cans. An old-fashioned icebox, a wood-burning stove. No fresh meat, unless it came from Japan, occasionally. We ate a lot of pheasant. My dad hunted. And Spam. I hated Spam.

147

Mother wrote to her mother in West Texas, requesting a "care package." Of Mexican food. Ashley's canned tortillas and Ashley's canned enchiladas. We ate like kings and shared with the compound. I had Mexican food for my 10th birthday party in Seoul, Korea, in 1948.

I was most fortunate!

7/12/94

Monday, I registered for Summer II—Special Therapies—10-12 M-Th, same as last semester. Will go in to work at 1 p.m. I set up files, ordered supplies and in general worked my tush off. Stayed till 6:30 tonight to get Robin ready for a meeting at HMFW tomorrow morning.

7/18/94

Now, do you think I'll become super-responsible? Well, maybe not. The happy medium would do. And I've done the responsible thing where the IRS and the foreclosure are concerned. I wrote to the collection agency and offered to make payments when I finish school and get a job.

And I was responsible for myself as far as the IRS is concerned. I told them I was a student and that my expenses were such that I couldn't quite make the $50 per month. I offered $35. We'll see. Why should I go ahead and bow to them and not take care of myself? I'm really proud of that.

Got a check from Terri today…$200. Also the TRC is back to paying $50 per week…So all that together is about $867 per mo which is about what I drew on UIC. I can make it.

Feeling sad tonight, too. Feel like crying, but I don't know why or about what. Just—sad. I have everything I need: food, shelter, clothing, friends and family…what else do I need?

"Love, power, freedom and fun." What is fun? What is freedom? What is power? And…what is love? Many kinds I have for friends/family, love

148

of God and my home and my country.

Much of the time I'm cheerful. I go through my day, feeling if not happy, at least content. Placid. Peaceful and maybe even serene.

And yet—at times, I feel this sense of—"Is that all there is?"

This will pass. It usually does.

8/23/94

Well, what a difference a week makes!

Mom and Dad came and went.

I registered for school.

It looks like this job is working, craziness and all. And we're moving closer to my house in Nov. I hope I'm still with them. I like my job. Miracle.

And, I asked the school to change my Creative Writing class that I'm teaching from Fri. afternoon to a morning and got Mondays at 9 a.m. Couldn't be better.

On a more "sour" note…My attorney Edwards told me that although my suit "can fly," it probably would be more trouble than it's worth. Even though the judge ordered him to pay, there were no consequences for him not doing so. There was nothing more I could do. I accept that and I give up. I've lived without his damn money. Maybe that's my "revenge"—that I can live without it. Wow!

I feel that something great is going to happen. I'm ready. Visit with Mom and Dad was the best ever. Tired, but a good tired.

I have grown, truly. About time!

8/31/94 Tuesday

First night of classes last night. Group counseling: We arrange our desks in a circle, as in group counseling. I like it. I can see everybody without turning around.

Anyway, Medical Aspects will also be interesting. Sam also said he was reminded that there were too many A's—"Scary." We

149

were reminded that we were overachievers.

I decided that life's too short to allow someone else to control my life—even from afar. We will no doubt be thrown together because of the baby...

Oh, yeah! I forgot to write that Lauri is pregnant. I'm going to be a grandmother in May! I'm so excited!

> Baby—what a sweet name!
> A new life
> Enters my life.
> A gift from my daughter
> And her husband.
> I had almost given up
> Ever being a grandmother.
> "Grandma"—I think not!
> The baby can call me
> "Mimi"—or whatever comes out
> Of that rosebud mouth.
> "Nana" would be fine, too.
> I could get really snooty
> And insist on
> "Grandmere"
> Or "Grand-Ma-Ma"
> And if the kid slips
> And calls me Grandma—
> I think that will be
> Just fine, too.

9/5/94 Monday

The people at TEC really annoy me. They act so damn superior, I think, that they have a job and I don't. Like it's my fault? That I'm "lazy" and don't want to work? And their damn Rules. You must follow the Rules. Line up. Wait for your name to be called. Fill out these forms. No, fill out these OTHER forms. You didn't fill it out completely, one smirks. I want to slap her silly.

I actually had a self-important civil servant shake her finger in my face, and tell me, "You didn't fill out the correct form."

I had a shame attack, and then I was angry. Who was this person to tell me what to do?

Well, she was the One With the Power.

She was the One Who Will Decide whether I get any money or not. Whether I can eat or not, or pay my house payment or not.

So I swallow my pride, get back in line and fill out the Correct Form.

10/3/94

Captured Moment

I am walking in the mall. It is early morning. My parents had called earlier. My mother said my father had walking pneumonia. Also said, almost as an aside, that his x-ray showed an incursion, right above the spot where his cancer had been cut from his lower right lobe six years ago.

Nobody said the words, "the cancer is back." After a few more banalities ("How's school doing?") where I wanted to shout, "For God's sake, look at what's really happening. Dad's cancer is back; it's going to kill him, can't you say it?"

Of course not. Sweep it under the rug with a few platitudes.

So I went walking—"life goes on"—and suddenly the word "abandonment" screamed in my head. Just when I think I'm resolving that issue with my father, he's going to be taken away from me...not by choice, he never left me by choice, but by the direct order of the U.S. Army...and I will really feel abandoned.

My breathing became rapid, my heart pounded, thudded, raced, and a total panic swept over me. The rational part of me said, "This is probably what a panic attack feels like."

It was.

151

Dialogue:

Me: Hey, Lupus.

Lupus: What?

Me: Don't you think you've done enough damage to my body? Not only to my body, but also to my mind and my spirit?

Lupus: I don't know what you're talking about. Haven't I left you alone for a while?

Me: Don't give me that. You thought you had me lulled into a false sense of security...until Thursday.

Lupus: So what happened Thursday to make you think this?

Me: The doctors think I have a heart murmur.

Lupus: Lots of people have heart murmurs. They're no big deal.

Me: Only those who don't already have lupus think they're no big deal.

Lupus: Didn't the doctors—both of them—tell you not to worry?

Me: Yeah, right. The message I got was, "Don't worry. Go on about your life, but if you get any chest pains or shortness of breath, go to the ER." That's not exactly reassuring. And they've scheduled tests for next month.

Lupus: If it were serious, they would have taken you in for tests right then.

Me: Yes, I guess so. It was only later, at the Lupus Seminar, that I read in a brochure that sometimes you can damage a heart valve, by putting some kinds of "nodes" on them, which causes a murmur. And the murmur is okay, unless infection sets in the grooves, and then "it becomes serious." I tell you, I don't have time for you!

Lupus: You don't have to get mad.

Me: Yes, I do. I never asked you into my life. You've just about taken over my life. Making me hurt, making me tired. I fought you with all I had, and by God, I won.

Lupus: Ha. You won the battle, but not the war.

Me: I refuse to accept that. The war is not over. We might have had an uneasy truce, but I didn't lose the war.

Lupus: I can still win, you know. You're weak right now. It would be easy.

Me: I'm just weak today. I pushed myself too far this week. I'm resting today. I'll be better tomorrow. So go away.

Lupus: Okay. Wait. But I'm still stronger.

Me: I'm not giving you any more power. I've done that—been afraid of you—too often. I have a secret weapon, you know.

Lupus: You can't keep secrets from me. I'm in your body.

Me: But not in my mind, or spirit. I have hope.

Lupus: What's hope?

Me: A way to deal with you; that you'll never take away from me.

Lupus: Hope? I don't think I know about that. I must consider this a while.

Me: You do that. Consider hope. It is much more powerful than you ever thought of being. Now, go away, or go to sleep—or do whatever it takes to keep you quiet.

Lupus: But your heart may be damaged...

Me: I don't know that, yet. I won't even consider that possibility today, thank you.

Lupus: Okay. I'm taking a nap now.

Me: Good. Make it a very long one. I'll call you next month with the test results.

Lupus: That's very considerate of you. Why?

Me: Because I respect you. The way I would want you to respect me. But I'm no longer afraid of you.

Lupus: You win. At least for today.

11/9/94

"You can't go home again"—how true. I went to the Brats reunion last weekend thinking—believing—I had no expectations. I accepted everybody right where they were...the Homecoming Queen, they tell me, has her head in the bottle. The

153

once handsome "star" of Linz Dependents High School is now dissipated and surly, who rarely speaks, and when he does, it's a mere mumble.

I wished some of my class had been there. I was treated with love and acceptance, as being a "fellow army brat," by those from the high school class. And I got to be "the kid" in a gathering of persons who were sixty or so.

I danced. I even drank a couple of German beers. Some kind of progress for me, since I had avoided parties, bars and dances where "drunks" would be there.

Another issue popped up, as I was packing to return home. I found myself throwing things into my suitcase. I thought, "I'm really angry, but I don't know why."

Was I terribly disappointed at the reunion?

I didn't think it was either. They didn't "fit."

It was only when I arrived home (thank God) and told my sponsor about my anger that I found out...

"One more time, you're having to leave some place," she said quietly.

And then I knew. All my life I had been saying good-bye...leaving my friends—my security—even if only for a little while.

I cried. Part of the crying was relief that I knew why I was angry. Part of the crying was for the young girl who wasn't allowed to cry at the time of separation. So I cry now.

11/12/94

Asthma?

Why am I still struggling with my health when I'm supposed to be in remission?

A trip to the ER early Thursday morning once again shows me that I'm vulnerable.

ASTHMA? Isn't it enough to have lupus, diabetes, high blood pressure—what the hell am I doing now with ASTHMA?

One of my earliest memories is of being under a "tent" of sheets. The vaporizer blowing steam in my feverish face. My mother is close by…she sometimes holds my hand. I survive but am prone to bronchitis every winter until I "outgrow it" at age twelve.

And now it sneaks back up on me. Am I doing something wrong? Should I have overextended myself as I did by going to my reunion at New Braunfels?

I can't stop living in order to live. I have plans for my future. And these plans do not include illness. I have been called stubborn; that's not all bad. Another word is perseverance. I know what is important to me, and by God's grace I will do it. I am doing it. I've been through much worse than this.

I have much to be grateful for. My friends and family. Their concern and help. My friend Virgie responding quickly to my 2:30 a.m. call when I barely could breathe the words: "I'm in trouble. Can you take me to the ER?" She came right away and stayed with me until it was determined I was stabilized.

My friend, Nancy, who called and gently scolded me for not calling her. I told her she had already taken me to the ER once; besides, she had to go to work that morning.

My friend, Joyce, who is walking her own walk with chronic pain. "Just" rheumatoid arthritis. Her calls help.

My bosses at work. I feel like I've let them down by being out. Just a couple of days, though, in 6 months. Not a bad record.

My brother, Bob, who told me not to worry about the apartment cleaning and laundry…he'd ask Jessie if she could do that for me on Sunday.

My fear is that something so trivial might kill me.

More than that, I might die before I've accomplished my tasks here on earth.

Surely God has a reason for my being here. Is it to finish school and work with others who are in pain—of any kind? It seems so. All the doors to that path have been opened. Am I supposed to write? If so, what should I focus on first? The story of my struggle with lupus? My army brat memoirs? My novel about the army wives during the years 1938-58? The "supernatural thriller Sabbath's Room" featuring my black cat Sabbath? Or something else that hasn't even presented itself yet?

Do I have the time?

Do I have the energy?

Would it be better/easier to quit school, find another husband and "have someone take care of me"?

What is my payoff? What am I doing now to get what I want? Everything.

But life keeps happening.

So I deal with it. The answers are there.

12/7/94 Wednesday

Pearl Harbor Day. Barely a mention in the news. How sad. I keep thinking of the words: "If it hadn't been for Pearl Harbor, we (Overseas Brats) would not have been where we were." Fascinating, how events transform lives.

I'm all stressed out. Bad day yesterday. Work was wild. Trying to get Robin to a 4:30 meeting. Ha. She was still on the phone. I left at 5:00. Couldn't do another thing.

Went to class (Group Counseling) and got there a bit late. Asked Sam about the 10 pt. article re: theory. If the name of the theory had to be mentioned. "Yes." Shit. The one I had picked didn't.

Also, the 5 questions for the final grade. Looked at the review sheet. Have to take another look at my answers. I probably did pretty good, anyway. Why do I worry about it? Because I always have.

Emotional class. Closure. Not a dry eye. Then on to Medical Aspects. When I left that class I went to the library to find an article...No luck. Left there around 9:30. Approaching my car, I noticed...felt...something was wrong.

Hell, my hubcaps were gone.

Pissed. Have only 1 hubcap left. Guess someone got scared away. Makes me mad that someone has to take from me. Lowlife scum.

Well, today is all I can handle. Today is only Wednesday and I have until Thursday night to revise my 5 questions and copy the article. Tonight is lupus support group Christmas dinner meeting. I'll take a salad.

God—help me to handle this stress. I need to take care of myself. I'm not feeling well. Chest congestion. A bit of a cough. Hope I don't start with the wheezing.

Have my regular lupus checkup on the 14th, lab work next Monday morning. Tired of all the medical crap. Tired of doctors, exams, meds...

Well, get off your butt and quit whining. Go to work and copy the damn article. Worry about the 5 questions tomorrow. Be more like Scarlett!

12/8/94

Woke feeling tired. Head sweat. Not bad, but a bit damp. Lupus support meeting last night. I was really tired before I went; came home from work and dozed for a few minutes.

Stopped by the store and got chicken wings. After the meeting (at which I ate turkey and salads and breads) I was really wiped out.

I worry that I might be getting a flare. That I might have to be hospitalized. Lose my job. Lose my apt.

I really do need a way to make enough money so I won't have to worry about "what if?" But if I feel too bad to work for it...it's a vicious circle.

God, help me. I'm scared. I don't think I'm so much afraid of dying, as I'm afraid I won't be able to have a quality of life.

Burned out? Quite possibly. I don't want to study any more. At least not today. I'm afraid I might not make good grades if I don't. So what's "good grades"? Well, A's of course. Can I just settle for passing? That would be okay. Lots of my classmates seem to be "just passing."

Hell, get up and get going and quit whining.

2/7/95

My Angel of the Highway

It's a miracle. God sent His holy angels to me tonight.

Stressed out day. Work a real challenge. Took off at 4 p.m. to go get chest x-ray and my car died right on Montgomery. Pulled into a parking lot. Tried to re-start. It did...so I went on to TCOM where I called Bob.

After the chest x-ray ($175 worth) I took my car to Bob at work. I told him I thought maybe I had pulled the key out a bit when it was attached by the spring-lock chain to my purse. We thought so...

Went on to class. Car was okay. Took my exam. Think I did okay. And started home.

The car stopped. I managed to pull to the median, put on my flashers, and pull out cellular phone....

And it's dead. Again. (I had taken it to the AT&T store yesterday and replaced the battery.) Then I found out they hadn't reactivated it. So I called 611 and raised hell.

They activated it tonight.

I went on to class. So here I am...Dead car. Dead phone.

A cold front is blowing in.

A car stops in front of me, backs up. Uh, oh, I think. God, please let it be a person I can trust. It's a woman.

She's in white slacks and white sweater. She identifies herself..."I'm an officer with the FW Police Dept." Then I see it's a police car.

She helps me by calling on her unit...the 800# for the towing service. We sit in her warm patrol car and talk.

She is a student, too. At UTA School of Nursing. She is divorced—13 years. She is an Air Force Brat. She asks me about my schooling, and praises me for having courage to do this...with lupus, yet.

I realize and say aloud..."I'm so glad I took my exam first."

She tells me my car probably has a fuel line problem.

She's truly an angel. She waits with me until the tow truck arrives. And it's a woman and her son...Margaret and Shawn Thomas.

They hook up my car and I get in. They bring me home and push my car into my carport. They tell me to call the 800# tomorrow and ask for them. They can take me to work on the way. Thank you, God!

The really strange part of all this is:
I never saw the car until I looked up and saw the back-up lights in front of me. I prayed, "God, please let it be someone I trust" and this woman in white steps out...identifies herself as a FW police officer—then I see that she's in a patrol car.

Also, when the tow truck comes, I am "busy" supervising them. We hug before she leaves. I turn my attention to the tow truck hookup, and when I look up again, she has gone. Vanished. So quickly.
I never saw her arrive, and I never saw her leave.
I know she was an angel.

Skeptics tell me I can call the FWPD and ask for her by name, and then I'd "really know."

I smile and say, "Why should I do that?"

6/18/95

It has been a tough last semester. Evidenced by no journal entries since Feb. I had no time or energy.

My schedule was: Work 40 hrs. per week, 8-5 M-F.

Classes M—5:30-6:30.

Tu-Th—8:30-9:50, home after 10:30.

Sat. Sun—practicum 10-2 CPC Millwood in Arlington and Wed/Thurs. at Excel. Corp. (practicum).

Plus projects. Dysfunctional Family Systems. The team's assessment of the movie: *When a Man Loves a Woman*—which earned our group a 105, plus personal praise for my writing the synopsis and speaking extemporaneously in front of my peers and professionals.

The other project was my family genogram. I sweat bullets over it. Up till the wee hours for 3 weekends, writing, drawing the diagram and praying it would get me an "A."

It got more than an "A." The instructor came past my desk before the next to final class and returned my chart and written history with a hushed, "It was wonderful!" Plus, she wrote at the end that I had a talent for writing and had accurately assessed my family's dysfunctions.

159

I made an A in the class.

Graduated with High Honors and in spite of the edict that we must wear black shoes, I wore red shoes. Hell with that, I thought. Red dress, red shoes.

I'm glad I did. That was the only way any of my friends and family could recognize me.

I also was a "graduate granny" since Joseph Douglas Landon entered the world on April 26. A moment to treasure when I held him. I think he knew his grandma.

Class reunion…June 7-9. What a hoot. Everyone is OLD. Except me, of course.

Wait till I get the video and addresses.

6/25/95

Thoughts on a Class Reunion—39 Years!

We meet again
Or is it the first time?
I gaze into a pair of eyes
And think, Who is this person?
My memory defeated,
My eyes drop to the (small) nametag.
I don't know this person.
But I say, "It's good to see you again," anyway.
And it is.
Good to see someone from our common era.
The Eisenhower, Pre-Sputnik, pre-Kennedy years.
We have a bond.
We know the same people, if not each other.
So we embrace fondly.
Strangers, yet not strangers.
Gray, balding, a tad heavier than we should be.
Wrinkles here and there—
Bifocals run rampant
Antacids are consumed discreetly

160

Post-dinner.
A few couples dance
Sedately
A couple attempts the Twist
And meekly give up,
Midway through.
Mostly, we visit,
Table to table,
Sitting more than standing.
Nobody drinks to excess
Just to show off.
I wonder why we are so
Happy to see each other.
These former classmates who were
Merely classmates, mostly, not
Close friends at all, like Sue and Norma
And Barbara and Frankie and me.
Just classmates.
Yet we embrace fondly
And seem genuinely pleased
With each other's accomplishments.
What will we do the next time we meet?
When we are more gray, more bald,
Slower to move?
We'll embrace fondly, we strangers,
Because we are of the same era.
We're survivors.

6/29/95

A lazy weekend. Didn't do much. But read and slept and slept and read. Went to church. That's about it. So I feel better. Go figure.

Saw the baby Tues. night. Precious. Fed him. He spit up. Burped him. He spit up. Saw him sleeping—just like Lauri used to, with his hands up over his head! Strong case for genetics, here.

161

I told Lauri she was a good mother. To trust her instincts. Took her 3 toy horses for the baby, of course. She likes them.

I was truly touched when I saw the afghan I had made for her YEARS ago is now in the baby's room.

Deadlines, always deadlines.

IRS—Aug. 15. School app. Aug. 1 (for Hampton funding). Always something.

I wish my video would come from the reunion.

7/15/95

Well, it came. I called Norma and said, "I'm watching a video of a bunch of fat old people. El Depresso."

Where have all the years gone?

Why has time treated so many of us so unfairly? And some of us haven't changed. Sue, Norma, Barbara, Frankie, Susan and me. Still friends.

Mom has been sick. Didn't go to the dr. Sick for 5 days with diarrhea. And I wonder why I never knew how to take care of myself!

God, I don't need to do any more compulsive shopping. Panties, okay, but not $150 worth of dress shoes. Even though I needed them, I can't afford it. Now I get to live in fear for the next payday.

A friend is in a depression and has been for some time. I recognize the signs—unpaid bills.

It seems to be a common thread among us...overspending, hoarding, fear of money, fear of no money...just all relating to fear.

8/4/95

Life is difficult. I do a lot of things I don't like that are tough...

It's discipline vs. self-will.

162

Getting old. Maybe that's what I'm angry about?
I don't like it.
Feeling old, left out of the main stream. No fun in my life.

8/6/95

All I know is, I'm feeling a bit depressed, and wondering what is causing it.

Maybe some of this depression is from my army brat years? A lot of old stuff is coming into my life.

My Linz reunion—my feeling so angry when I left New Braunfels.

8/8/95 Tuesday

Feeling crummy. Ache like I have the flu.

Is this a flare? I'm scared. Angry. I don't like having to go to work, anyway. Even when I'm sick. I can't afford to use up my PTO time.

I need to get my taxes together and send it off.

Terri wants us to go to Europe. Well! Wouldn't that be nice? I don't know how I can afford it. Please show me how, God.

We could join a college tour. That would be cheap. Probably more fun and interesting, too.

I feel really strange…not really sick. Just "blah."

I feel like my hands are weak. My leg muscles…not pain. Just aches.

I'm pretty tired of this. Is it my meds?

Do something today about this…If I have to go to the dr.

3/11/96 Monday

Found THE book! *Military Brats: Legacies of Childhood Inside the Fortress* by Mary Edwards Wertsch.

I had been looking for this for about two years! Out of print, out of luck. So I tried Half Price Books.

How I found it was a miracle...

After church Sunday, I convinced myself that I really need a new red suit. My current red suit is really worn. Couldn't find one at Morton's or at Burlington. As I was leaving, I thought, "Hey, there's the Half Price Bookstore; I haven't looked in this one yet." Also need to get a German-English phrase book for when Terri and I go to Germany.

Which I did. And looked for the sociology section...No sociology section. "Now where else could it be?" I thought. But hey, here's a clearance corner...Might find something there I'd love to have.

Now, God knows I'm short. I never look on high shelves; usually start at least at eye level. But this time, I looked up as I entered the clearance corner—and saw only the spine of a book that said—in blue letters on white background—"Military Brats."

My heart stopped. Surely not. Surely this is another book by the same title...but no, correct author. And correct subtitle. And the $20 book was now $2.96.

Wow! I clutched it to my heart and breathed a prayer. Thank you, God.

Silly to go on about this, but I believe this was a "God deal." It was just too much of a coincidence.

And the book validated me. All the years of being a Brat...confirming my feelings.

4/6/96

Terri and I are going to Germany and Austria.

We leave June 5, return 16th. Will stay with Lisa in Munich, sightsee and then go to Austria. A couple of days. Then to Paris. Terri's heart's desire.

Had a garage sale on 1st April. Made $165 and put it in savings right away.

God is good.

4/21/96

My 58th birthday. How did I get here so fast? Old. Older. I find myself worrying about my memory. CRS. My waistline has vanished. Wrinkles cropped up. Horrid liver spots on my hands.

Despite my efforts—my denial that these things will occur... they have.

"Youthful exuberance" is what my boss wrote on my birthday card.

Compliments of "You don't look your age" abound.

I have:

Good and loyal friends. Fine and wonderful children. A roof over my head, with trees, wind chimes, soothing music any time I want, health (so far so good.) A planned trip to Austria...a lifelong dream of returning to my favorite place in the world.

A God who loves me and who has sustained me through all my adversities as I have survived:

A military brat childhood, my father's absences punctuated by brief but benign tyrannies; two miserable marriages endured as long as humanly possible, then broken, to be followed by years of financial insecurity, loneliness that could not be filled by affairs and life threatening illness(es).

I have endured more than some, not as much as others.

I have not yet lost a parent to death. My children are alive and healthy. I have a grandchild, nieces, and a large family to call upon.

In spite of my fears of becoming a bag lady, I have never missed a meal, found myself without shelter or without assurances from family and friends that I'll be all right.

Today, I'm okay.

Today, I'm 58.

I'm blessed.

6/11/96

Trip to Europe…We return on Dad's birthday.
*I called him from the airport in Newark and wish him a happy birthday.
He is very faint. I feel very sad.*

6/30/96

My parents' 59th wedding anniversary. Mom called about how Dad is doing.

We both cry. Finally.

Both had been trying to "out brave" each other.

July 4 weekend…

I go visit Dad. Am shocked at his appearance. He was in the recliner, in his pajamas. And looked so gaunt. Like a concentration camp inmate. His eyes and mouth seem too big for his skull. He is very weak. Listless.

I feel he is withdrawing. Partly due to his illness (talking is very tiring) partly because he *is* withdrawing.

I feel so sad.

Mother says his arm is tingling now, an indication that the tumor is pressing on the artery. He started chemo again.

If the cancer doesn't kill him, the treatments will.

7/26/96 2:40 a.m.

A dream woke me. I dreamed my grandpa was dying. I saw him—looked as thin as Dad, lying on a counter in a corner, next to a sink, so he could vomit in it.

I am bringing him food (cake?). He doesn't want it.

Later, I hear he died. That he was calling out to his dad: "Wait for me."

I wake up. Wonder if it's my dad.

166

Half-ass analysis: Grandpa was due to my looking at Woody's letter ending with "give Grandpa and Grandma my regards."
I have thought Dad looked like Grandpa at the end of his life.

8/11/96 Sunday

Woke feeling bad. Tired, achy. After a good night's sleep. Short of breath. I finally do the flow meter and guess what? It's 175. That's worse than it was 2 years ago at Christmastime.

Let's see: Stressors are: I negotiated a raise, got it, finished asset inventory at work, had exam in class; studying for finals; pushing thoughts of my father dying back and away; worrying about my mother; got all my paperwork done and sent off to UNT; wonder if going to school is such a good idea after all. Money problems, as usual; pissed off at Doug; I didn't get to see my grandchild very often and when I do, it's a real stressor. Beating up on myself because I'm not doing better—better than what? Been missing church and Al-Anon, due to demands on my health.... I don't like taking care of myself; everybody seems to have a boyfriend but me (what's wrong with me?)

Enough stressors? Add the drive to classes in 5 p.m. traffic.

Well, hell, no wonder I feel bad! I'm overdue for an asthma attack. At least.

Worry about ol' Lupe saddling up and riding through my body again. Has she started already?

I'm grateful for: My trip to Europe, my family, my friends, what health I have left, school, work, my co-workers, my recovery, God in my life, even when I didn't think of Him; He thinks of me and loves me. My father—that we, today—have a relationship at last. That I'm not angry with him any more.

9/4/96

I've been putting this off.
Dad died on Wed. Aug. 21. I had been there the weekend before.
He deteriorated right in front of my eyes.

167

Friday, he was able to get up and go to the bathroom.

Saturday, he collapsed when we tried to help him into the wheelchair.

The three of us ended up in a heap.

Dad kept repeating, "Oh, me."

He became incontinent on Saturday.

Mom called in "reinforcements" who could be with her 24 hours a day.

He was coherent only half the time. Looked like any little old man in a nursing home. Teeth out, unfocused eyes, no meat on his bones. Thinking about and calling out to unseen persons.

Like his own mother. Hallucinating?

He said, looking over at the corner of the room, "Hello, Mother."

I know she came to take him home with her.

He seemed to give in. Not give up, but he gave in. He recognized me at his bedside.

I told him Bob and Gary were coming. Soon. He said, "I'm proud of my boys."

I left on Sunday. Reluctant to go. Called my brothers. Told them it looked bad. They'd better hurry and change their reservations from Sept. 6 to Friday.

They did.

But it was too late.

Mom called me on Wed. 21 at 7 a.m. He expired at 5 a.m. in his sleep.

Thank God he had no pain.

Thank God he didn't linger long, unable to live *or* die.

The funerals were hard. Taps and the rifle volleys. The honor guard, stiff and at attention. Dedicated. The flag. The memorial service, where I spoke.

My brothers crying their hearts out at the funeral home. I'm grateful they didn't see him as I had—all helpless and gaunt. Not at all the Dad we knew.

I'm numb. Fatigue sets in on that Monday, as if the day were 2 days long. Faced with the long drive home to Fort Worth on Tuesday.

How did I do all this?

I cried for my father.

I cried over my mother's grief and worried that I might lose her, too. She experienced nosebleeds as her stressor.

I just quit thinking and went on autopilot.

I'm grateful that I healed our relationship.

I no longer felt abandoned, even though my father's leaving was, at this time, for sure, permanent.

But I'll see him again.

And he still lives in my heart—and in my head.

Thanks, Dad. For all you taught me.

I love you.

10/20/96 Sunday

Bummed. Have a bad attitude. Sick and tired of being sick.

Cough. Sneeze. Cough again. Since last week.

Hate this HMO crap. Went to the dr. on Tues or Wed at the clinic. A woman. She put me on antibiotics and inhalers and nasal sprays. Not better on Friday, so I call in…see another dr.

He is an arrogant little bastard. Implies I'm a hypochondriac, but orders a chest x-ray anyway. Well, of course! I'm thinking about changing doctors again. Go back to Dr. Marsh and Dr. Anderson.

Bad mood persists thru today. Need to study—can't—need to clean—can't. Need to write—can't—need to go to office and do my Excel exercises for class—can't. Shit.

Thinking about giving up on school. Whine a lot to Sabbath. Who doesn't care. She's just being a cat.

I haven't had a weekend. I haven't felt good yet.

My ribs hurt from coughing so hard. Or maybe I have pneumonia? God forbid that this doctor should know that.

When I'm down physically, I'm down emotionally—and mentally and spiritually.

Oh, I almost forgot God.

I'm glad He doesn't forget me.

169

Nothing is really wrong, right this minute.

Right now, nothing is happening. No exams, no need to do my computer stuff right now.

So what did I get done? Well, I paid my bills today.

I went to class yesterday.

10/31/96

Trick or Treat!

Halloween.

Found out last Friday that ol' Lupe is back. In my pleura. "Lupus Pleuritis" is officially diagnosed. After all the howling I did at the clinic—the x-ray showed it.

Dr. apologized. Yeah, right. I was so shocked and scared. I cried. I asked for my regular doctor, not an intern.

No, I demanded *to see my regular doctor. He assured me this is just a flare. But I feel so tired. Like I did before. The main thing is to keep from getting pneumonia. So I'm on antibiotics and high doses of prednisone.*

At least I'm not hurting really bad. And the coughing has almost stopped.

But I'm still angry that it took so long to realize I'm having a flare. And I'm just plain mad that it's back!

Lupe must be pleased. She waited and softened me up, lulled me into a false sense of security. Then, when I returned from Europe, going to Mom's a couple of times and starting school again at Denton and *TCJC—*

I've made arrangements to finish the semester, though. Too close to quit. I'll pass and then lay out next semester. So yesterday: I went to work. As usual. Didn't miss any except 2 days in the last two weeks. Still have 90 hours PTO. I can always take short-term disability if possible. And I can't get fired because of it.

I trudge on.

But damn, I'm still mad.

I need to look at the possibility of not going back to school next semester.

11/20/96

Still feeling kind of tired. So grateful that I've dodged the bullet, though.

I'm almost glad I'm not going back to school next semester. It will be cold, dark, dreary—the long drive and the studying—I don't need that at this time in my life.

Am I wrong in thinking I don't need any more stress than necessary at my age? After all, I have to be realistic.

What are my needs?

My needs are being met. Except for companionship. It would be nice to have someone wonder where I am at night, someone to pick me up at the car dealership. Someone to carry things up the stairs. To be there for me, to confide in.

I know I have these things with my friends. But they're not always with me, and I have to ask. I've done that. I know all I have to do is ask for help...but...I'm lonely. For the first time, I don't treasure my independence. I hear about others who rely on their husbands—who do things together—and I feel lonely.

1/12/97

Not much change. Have a bad upper respiratory infection—again—got an antibiotic. Will take it for 2 weeks then have blood work done at Dr. Marsh's. She doesn't think it's lupus.

I wonder.

Life sucks. And my attitude right now.

I'm supposed to go to the Petroleum Club on Monday night with Judy and Joyce. I have my dress all ready. My spirit is willing. My body is not.

It's snowing. I'm warm, semi-well. I still have lights and heat and food. And family and friends. This, too, shall pass.

But I want it to hurry up.

Serene. I sit in my chair beside the window. Listening to classical music.

What I had envisioned years ago—a room with sun, music, books, flowers.

So the flowers aren't real! And the music comes from a borrowed system. I still have the sunlight thru the trees and plenty to read.

Easter. A rebirth. I feel very well, for a change. I have cleaned my apt. already this morning. Even re-hung the wreath on the front door. It kept falling off. So, of course, I needed another wreath. Until it occurred to me—DUH—that what I needed was a longer nail to hang it on!

Three whacks with a hammer on a long nail did it. Amazing.

I have plans to go see Katie at her birthday party at 2:00. Got her some Barbie stuff. I don't know if she has a "Ken" but there's a "groom" in the set. Just like me—looking for a Ken.

Work is still amazing. I'm going to get a raise and promotion to AAIV, which starts at 11.48 per hr. That's about $200 a month more. I'm trying not to spend it all before I get it.

Besides that, I get a $350 refund from the IRS. It seems the minute I surrendered my finances and asked for help, things changed.

God works in mysterious ways.

Have Easter basket all ready for Joseph. Made it myself. A blue bunny standing in the middle of the basket with large plastic eggs filled with candy all around. Plus a rubber duck for bath time. Need to see him…

Mom is going to Terri's Tuesday. Wish I could go. But that's not possible now. Later this summer, when it's scorching, here, I can go.

4/29/97

Really exhausted. Dr. M. says she'll check my thyroid and sed rate. Could be I'm beginning a flare.

Could be I'm low on thyroid.

Much stress…lots of work. Not any strength left for play.

Play? What's that?

I had playtime with Joseph at his birthday party. 2 years old! He loved the tool set I gave him. Knows how to use the screwdriver.

Work is a bitch. Too much. No raise yet. After all that work. Ungrateful s.o.b. I work for. He makes me mad. Wants me to be perfect on software when he can't do it. What's wrong with this picture?

5/3/97 Saturday

Still tired. Went to Dr. M on a Monday. Complained of fatigue, weight, sleepiness, and heaviness in chest. Waking as tired as I was before sleep. She took blood tests on thyroid and suggested I might be starting to flare.

Hell. That means more cortisone. But I'm not there yet. Tests haven't come back yet.

Went to Mayfest Thurs. night. Had enough energy for that! Symphony played 1812 Overture with fireworks and cannon.

I thought of Dad. Figured he was directing the cannon.

Is it lupus?
Always a specter
In the back of my mind.
Is it here, again?
Of course, it never really
Went away.
It was just asleep.
Or lurking around the corner,

Waiting its chance
To snare me again.
God, take this from me
If it is Your will.
I cannot imagine
That You want me ill.
Maybe You just want me
To learn some lessons.
The lessons are hard, God.
Harder than any others
I've learned.
So far.
Give me grace, Lord,
To live with this enemy
Each day.
Today, I'm (semi) okay.
Not as energetic
As I'd wish,
Tired of being tired, God.
Dragging myself around
Is tiresome.
I really try to rest
(Foreign word that it is.)
But I have to work
(Thank You for the strength to do that)
And I want to play
(And sometimes I manage to do some of that.)
So all in all, I guess,
I'm where I'm supposed to be.

9/20/97

Dreamed I was in Austria last night. Castle on the hill. We were going to climb to it. We got there. Then came an avalanche. We sought refuge inside the sturdy castle. The avalanche began by a cracking of the ice in the mountain.

174

Does this mean? I am a "stronghold"? Sturdy castle? I have the strength (maybe not physically) to withstand the onslaught (avalanche) of emotions? Of events?

Certainly there have been events...the boiling cauldron of mergers...uncertainty of my job...despite the fact that my boss assured me I will have a job. And my long-awaited raise.

My work is more than satisfactory.

Maybe that's one reason I withdrew from school. Besides the stress factor. I don't need the admiration of others any more. The remarks of "Well, I certainly admire you." I know I am loved for who I am, not what I do.

Also dreamed about crying. Buckets and oceans of tears. (The avalanche?) I know I haven't grieved over my father's death. How am I supposed to grieve over someone I didn't know? Over someone I was so angry with for so long, for seemingly abandoning me? My head knows that's not true.

But the heart of the little girl doesn't believe it. Maybe I need to grieve for what could have been? I had a part in that relationship, too. And I could only resist my father's attempts to show love to me. "Brat" is my middle name!

10/25/97 Saturday morning

Well, I took a giant step yesterday. I emailed HR about my "non-raise." Explained my concern that it was granted in June and I will have another boss soon, due to the merger, so this raise will be forgotten, with nobody taking responsibility for implementing it.

Maybe it would be "Christmas money." I could use it then. And put some in savings. And have my computer upgraded.

Dammed inconvenient not having a CPU at my workstation. IT will move Hao's to mine on Monday. Or install our software on the "old, unused" pc and move it. I need to pray for the thief who stole my computer last week. I walked in the door, set my purse down and reached down to power up the computer. And it was gone! I called IT to see if they had "borrowed" it for some reason. I called Security and reported the theft. Amazing.

11/16/97 Sunday a.m.

No raise yet. Tuesday I'll file a grievance.

Cleaned closet yesterday. It's all in order now, except for things that need pressing.

12/7/97

Pearl Harbor Day. I think of my trip to Hawaii and remember seeing Pearl Harbor. How very narrow it is. The sight of a ship approaching with its men standing at ease on the decks. A real awe-inspiring sight.

And "if it weren't for Pearl Harbor, none of us would have had the experience of being an Overseas Brat."

I GOT MY RAISE!!!!

At last!! Proud of myself for standing up for myself. Feeling powerful.

I'm tired today. Put up the tree, etc. No wonder I'm tired.

Achy. Wet weather hurts. Arms, mostly. Feel congested in pleura. Sort of twinge-y.

Old age or lupus flare? Or the beginnings of a cold? Wait and see.

1/26/98 Monday p.m.

Holidays over…at last back to journaling. Feeling somehow out of synch, today.

Rested all weekend and hated it. It's not like me to do nothing

Job is going well. Stress almost gone. Nonexistent, really. Some days I fight boredom. I'm so well-organized. Love my new area….

Two concerns today—

1. Heard where Gordon from our lupus support group had died. Of lupus. I'm going to the funeral tomorrow at 2 p.m.

2. Called Patty B to ask her if she was going and talked to her husband.

Patty has had renal failure. Is on dialysis, will go next for a transplant. Double whammy! Fear set in.

What are these 2 incidents telling me? That I'm next? Or doomed? I don't think so. That I need to watch my health? Well, duh. That's what I did all weekend. That I need to "live it up"? I do know I need to pray for them both, and their families. And ask God to keep me in the palm of His hand.

4/10/98 Friday a.m.

Took the day off. Planned it. Will also have Monday off. Wow.

I see I haven't journaled in a long time. No excuse. Just haven't done it. I feel I have grown so much lately. I had a paradigm shift.

My job is stretching me. Not stress-wise, but learning how to handle stress. I've learned I can stand up to a boss and not get into fear when he goes ballistic. I know he's as frustrated as I am, or more, with the changes the merger has made.

Well, it's 10:49 a.m. and I'm still in my gown. I've made my bed, done the dishes, cleaned the refrig and emptied the trash baskets.

Today I plan to get some impatiens, go to the store for coffee and paper towels and just get frozen things for dinners. I've decided I'm just wasting fresh salads, fruits and vegs. Because I don't eat them before they spoil.

Then I'll read this afternoon and pay bills. And tonight is Stations of the Cross at 6 p.m. I feel so blessed, with my family and friends and work. If I have to go to work in Las Colinas, I'll pray about it. Keep my options open. I don't have to decide today.

6/19/98

Father's Day tomorrow.
My father is gone...again.
And this time he's not coming back.
The Supreme Commander issued orders
And he went immediately.
My adult mind tells me
My father died.
My little girl's heart, however,
Still wishes he were home.
My father was my strength—
He taught me, by his actions,
To be flexible.
To go without question.
Move here and there with no complaints.
Mother, God love her,
Resisted. Or so it appeared to me.
She moved, but not willingly.
She, too, sought some stability,
And resisted, even though unconsciously,
Every change.
I learned from them both.

6/19/98

Class Reunion's over. Still processing.
Learned something:
I was different, says Sue. I had remarked that Lawton folks accepted military people more than any other city. But Sue said, "No, that's not right. You were different from the other army kids. You made an effort to belong."

Staying with Sue in her home left me to long for another bedroom, a bigger kitchen/dining area. But that means more $$. Can I do it? And still go and do what I want and not worry so much about every penny?

God will have to tell me. I don't have a clue. OK, God: My wish list:

A larger kitchen with windows and room to sit in.
Dining area a bit larger.
View from kitchen into living area, for TV
Extra bedroom
Extra bathroom
Covered parking
Sunlight/shade/modern, yet not too.
My own heat/air
Downstairs
No sliding glass doors.
Pets allowed
Beige carpet. Tiled bath floors.

8/24/98

Okay, God, are you laughing? Well, 10 ½ out of 12 ain't bad. Decided to move downstairs, right here. Not only did I get the above list, I also have a fireplace and a teeny little patio area outside the sliding glass door. Actually, I now have 3 exits—kitchen door, front door and sliding glass door.

The maintenance guys were great with the move. They even packed some stuff!

Took off Friday, Mon and Tues.

All that's left are the guest room and the closets. I can't believe I'm so comfortable already.

Oh, yes, I have a new couch, too. Even wrote a check for it. Never thought I could do that.

God is soooo good.

So much good stuff lately. I'm so grateful for my health. Must remember to take good care with myself so I won't get a flare.

Nancy and Joyce left on a cruise Friday. Just wait till they get back and see my place!

4/9/99 Friday

Been really bad about writing in my journal. Lots happened.
Got out from under the job that I had.
Got a new job at the downtown location.
It's really busy.
I know I need to lighten up on myself. I'm trying to do 2nd grade work while I'm in the 1st grade.
Dream one night:
I was having a baby. 3 year (3 hour?) labor. It is a girl. Named her—and very emphatic about it—"Rachel Elizabeth."
Must mean something. Darned if I know what.
I am serious about wanting to never have to answer to anybody ever again. Never having to show up with my butt in a chair at 8 a.m. every weekday.
I'm too old for that shit. I also need to make enough money for my "old age." Right?

4/11/99 Sunday

To church or not to church? Why have I been absent? Stress. But one would think that stress would drive me to church! Not me. When it's tough, I don't go. When it's not tough, I go? But it has been tough since Christmas!
First the knee surgery. Back up—first the knee injury I sustained while moving downstairs...then company, then Christmas, then the job stress, then the change in job, then the new job stress...it's always something. Get back to church!

4/11/99

Dream:
I am to make a speech.
I don't know what the subject is. I don't know what I'll say. But I'll be okay. Two kids have left me without a car. We will be late. We are at some mountain lodge and there are avalanches

180

around us. I see them...Two—one comes very close. In fact, we almost get buried, but it stops short. On to the speech. I am angry that the 2 kids left me without a car. I have gone home and changed to my PJ's...do I have to go speak in them? I need a car to go home and change before I speak. Suddenly, I am ready, dressed for the speech. I am wearing blue.

Also—I'm working on a computer...I am seeing the results of my "send" show as blips on a map of the world...Africa, England, New Zealand, etc. I am pleased.

Maybe that has to do with writing?

4/17/99

I dreamed last night I was going to college. University of North Texas. Was going to be late. Others went on without me while I searched for my schedule. Much to my surprise, I wasn't enrolled. By the time I got to UNT, class would be over. I spoke to a bearded man who seemed to be in charge. He said he would check into it. By that time, I realized I didn't want to go, after all.

Was it God? I know the "late to class" means I have lessons to learn...but I'm willing to show up. Late? Probably means I'm learning late in life.

Previous dream of 3 months/years dream...something highly significant will happen to me then.

5/1/99

May Day. Remembering Austria with the May Day Parades of Communists, squeaky shoes, us kids at the school windows, laughing. Our teachers horrified.

Korea, May Day—4th grade...May Pole Dance. I borrowed a white dress. Didn't have one. Ticked about it. Why didn't I have a white dress? Probably because it would have been impractical— too easy to get dirty. Mom was right.

A dream...Dad gave me a cross...like my pewter one.

181

I asked Mom today when she called if he ever gave me a cross when I was a kid. She said he couldn't remember that he did. Just now noticed: "A cross" could be I feel he is "cross" with me? Authority—my boss? Or is he trying to get something across to me?

11/6/99

Rash on upper arm. Got up at 2 a.m. Watched TV a while. Disturbed Sabbath. Right side of head hurts again. Above ear. Residual from shingles. Damn. Some part of me is always hurting or in a rash!

4/8/2000

I Quit My Job!

Sabbath died March 20. I grieved before she died, so when I woke up and she was next to me, cold and still, I accepted it. Twenty years, my companion. Gone. I miss her dreadfully. Don't think I'll get another cat.

Work sucked so bad I'm taking FMLA. May have shot myself in the foot, but at least they can't fire me and I'll have 3 weeks plus short-term disability till I feel better. Stronger. More sane. Will seek counseling. First through EAP, then referral.

So, I prayed for some time off so I could write. So why am I not writing today? Tired. Need to take at least this weekend to do nothing. Am still in my pajamas at 11 a.m. Bed not made. Just reading the paper, drinking coffee, nothing planned for today. I am having a hard time with that. I am so "busy" oriented. Don't know how to "do nothing." Does that make me lazy?

I think not. Taking care of myself, this minute, means doing nothing. Rest. That's not laziness.

I'm still in shock from Friday…when I gave notice of my intent to take FMLA. Then I came home, changed clothes and lay down on the couch with the quilt over me. Slept from 11 a.m. to 2:00 p.m. Woke up, ate some lunch, watched *Oprah*. My former boss called from the office. Could I meet the temp Sat. at 1 p.m. to show her what I do? Did that. Temp is wild-eyed by the time I finish. "Do you do all this, every day?" I said, "And more."

She left due to prior commitment. I stayed and sorted all my paperwork, putting sticky notes/instructions on all the stacks. Then I came home and slept an hour. Woke just in time to meet Joyce and Nancy at Uncle Julio's for Nancy's birthday. They have been so supportive thru this…as have my family.

Feeling a tinge of fear. How will I manage on 60% of my income? On $480 every two weeks? I have enough food. Bought $95 worth of rice, beans, canned goods on Friday.

Am I tired or depressed? Both. So I don't need to kick myself. Enjoy Easter!

Undated

My eyes are full of unshed tears.

Tears over Dad's death, still. Sabbath's death. Loss of my job, even though temporarily. Loss of self-esteem. Loss of spirit.

I will never again get myself into a job where my spirit is crushed daily!

4/15/00 Saturday

My first week of freedom has passed.

6/22/00 Thursday

Diagnosis by Dee Carter: "Acute Stress Disorder." DUH!

Diagnosis by Philip Wilson—"Major Depression." HUH?

Hell, now I *feel* depressed! Asked him: When did this start? How do I get better? Of course, the answers are: I've been depressed most of my life. Really began with my 2nd divorce and Dad's death and Sabbath's death and job loss…ARRGGHH.

Okay, need to grieve so many things.

183

6/23/00 Friday 7:15 a.m.

Got a good night's sleep. No 2 a.m. tossing and turning. Dreamed, but no nightmares. Leaving to go to Mom's in the a.m. Early, of course.

So much on my mind.

Can't possibly work under this depression. I have no concentration. Funny, I can write with no problems. But I would have—did have—problems following orders because my mind was in a fog.

Couldn't cope with that job a day longer. Workers Compensation wanted a "date of injury." I had been injured from the first day. My spirit was broken, crushed; not being treated as a person of worth and dignity took its toll.

It was time for me to get out. To find nurturing, acceptance and respect. I couldn't get it there. I found it within.

I am worth more than my job.

My job today is just to breathe. To function. To put one foot in front of the other. To grieve over losses. All my losses. Good, bad or indifferent. Wrote a "Grief and Loss" list:

My lost childhood, my father's absence, my lost friends, my marriages, bad as they were; my other relationships, bad as they were; my health, my children, my self-esteem, my loss of income.

My life was not supposed to be this way. It's not what I had planned.

I had planned to be a good wife and mother with a loving husband, and a comfortable life. Well, 2 for 2 isn't bad. I think I was a good wife—I did all the right things. I know I was a good mother.

6/26/00 Monday a.m.

Home from Mom's. Tell her we're going to give her a reception for her 80th birthday.

Brothers irritated me. Male bonding crap. Loud—each trying to outdo the other.

I told them of my major depression. Bob couldn't even respond. Gary nodded. Said probably started with my first divorce. I didn't tell him I think I've been depressed most of my life. Just now all hitting at once.

I'm grateful I have this time to do nothing but grieve and get well.

Update last night. Tired but not able to sleep. Asthma again. When I lie down, I hear the wheeze and rattle.

Talked to Terri. She starts to cry. I tell her I'm really okay. Just depressed as hell. She worries I might get sick again.

I assure her I'm taking good care of myself. She will help me any way she can…$$ and with getting a condo. Start looking.

Today I need to call Liberty Mutual re: the check I received.

Is this for real? Has my claim been approved? Or is this just "back wages"? Go to the bank. Deposit check, anyway.

Grieve. Let it go.

I hadn't planned on marrying alcoholics. I hadn't planned on having a chronic illness. I hadn't planned on losing jobs. I hadn't even planned on working!

6/28/00

Stuck

I am stuck
In a hole
That has no bottom.
I want out.
I want some energy.
I want, I want, I want!
And I want it now.
Lord, give me strength
To see this THING thru
And let me climb out
Of this hole

185

That has no bottom.
I'm not depressed, I say.
I'm not crying
Or feeling weepy
Or sad.
But my body says, "Yes,
You are depressed.
Rest."
Rest, exercise. Eat well.
Sleep. Don't sleep.
Can't sleep.
Sit here and meditate.
Get up and clean the house.
Eat. Don't eat.
At least, don't eat
Because you're stressed.
Shower, Dress, Makeup
Put on your face
For the world to see.
I'm fine, I reply—
They say I'm looking great!
They don't see the dead eyes,
The don't see my insides
My insides that are full of
Anger, resentment, grief
Anxiety knotting me up.
I want to lose weight.
I don't want to add another stressor
To my already overflowing plate
Of depression.
So I won't deprive myself
Of chocolate, at least.
My brain has all but expired.
Confusion reigns. Short-term memory
Shot all to hell.
Mix up appointments.

Make a big, huge error in my checkbook.
Can't hold a thought
More than a nanosecond.
My brain needs help!
Not enough serotonin.
I'm medically ill.
My brain is sick.
My brain is not my mind.
My brain is a physical
Part of my body.
A part that isn't working
Quite right.
Synapses don't connect right?
Due to lupus?
Chronic illness
Has built up toxins
In my brain.
Telling me I need to sleep.
Or not.
How to rid the toxins
Without destroying the brain?
That's a dilemma
I thought I'd never have.
"Stoic." My mind says.
I'm stoic.
My mind is not my brain.
My brain is just the engine
For my body.
My mind is the driver.
My mind sometimes takes
A detour
Where I am lost for a while.
I don't like this detour.
It's not very scenic.
Even if it were scenic,
I wouldn't enjoy it.

187

Because I want back
On the road
To recovery.
My mind tells me lies.
My brain stores them.
From birth—or before—
I have thought myself:
Stupid. Unworthy.
Less than. Different.

Let's look at stupid. No way am I stupid. Not knowledgeable about a lot of things, but not stupid. As I was watching a movie on TV, it showed a girl studying in the lunchroom. My thought? "I don't know as much as a high school kid."

Maybe not math, chemistry or engineering, but I can beat any high school kid today in English, history and geography.

I'm not stupid. Just haven't learned some things yet. Bet I could pass those things if I wanted to. I just don't see the need for math, chemistry, engineering right now.

Why did I bother?

It was nothing that I did or didn't do, to be treated callously. To be neglected, to be tossed aside…for someone younger, prettier, and—not so smart!

I didn't cause it, I can't control it, I can't cure it. Let it run its course.

I *will* pull out of this hole.

7/3/00 Sunday evening

God, please help me with my writing. Show me what to sell and where…show me what to write and when.

Give me the energy to create.

Looking back at my last job—I was sick then. After I transferred to the downtown office I got the shingles. I had headaches. I had upset stomachs.

I couldn't do anything right.

I was too well to work there. I realized my spirit was being crushed. I was treated badly. And I didn't deserve to be treated that way. None of it was my doing.

Why have I always felt that when bad things happen, it's my fault?

When good things happen, it's just luck?

I worked hard for that good luck!

Cry, dammit. I'll feel better and heal quicker if I can grieve.

It's buried so deep—I have pushed all my sorrows down into that bottomless hole; I fear I'll never get them out.

Maybe that's what this hole is for? Why I'm in it. I might be in this dry well...so I can examine what is at the bottom and deal with it.

I see many issues at the bottom of the well. One by one, I pick them up and examine them. Here's my father's "abandonment." Here's my grief over leaving friends and a place I loved. Here's my first marriage, broken to pieces by his actions, not mine. Here's my second marriage—same as above.

Here's lupus wallowing around in the mud. Dormant now, it is capable of striking at any time. Sneaky damn disease that robbed me of several years. Here are the multiple conditions resulting from the lupus meds and making my body and brain toxic. Here are the doctors who didn't pick up on and treat me for lupus in the first three years of my search.

Here are the jobs I lost, due to lupus. None of them was my fault. I was so ill I should have been able to stay at home.

Here is Social Security, HMOs and prescription drugs. Not going to manage at my age now, must wait till I'm 65 before SS will do me any good, and I can work all I want, then. Here's my disability claim and workers comp claim.

Here's my pride—bent all to hell.

Here's my spirit—crushed, but salvageable.

What should I put in the wooden bucket first, to send to the top?

I wish I could get in the bucket first and have someone pull me up.

189

But I must deal with these issues here, and then climb up and out, myself.

Let it begin today.

7/8/2000 Saturday

Mom called this morning. We talked about her upcoming reception. She's already bought a lavender dress for it. Of course.

We set the time for 5-7 p.m. Light hors d'oeuvres. Order cake from Nadlers in SA.

I wanted to tell her about my depression, but didn't. She doesn't need to know, I reason.

Am I right?

Does it matter?

I need to get on a schedule, now that I'm not working. It might make me feel better.

Or do I need to feel better and then get on a schedule?

7/10/00

Too many thoughts trying to intrude. Need to call the realtor who called me back Sat. and start looking at condos.

Terri is coming in from Cancun the Thursday before Mom's birthday event. We'll look at condos then.

Still no word about short-term disability. Need to fill out the form that w/c sent me and mail it in. Had stomach problems yesterday. I understand that's part of the depression.

Need to start weeding things out. Giving to Goodwill—need to see when they pick up.

Got the "Don'twannas."

Am I putting too much on my plate right now?

Can I handle all this?

It might help pull me out of this....

Or it might make me worse?

Ask my shrink.

History of depression: First dx with "adjustment disorder"
—in the 90s at Family Center. Right after lupus episode.

Time passed. I worked, didn't work, went to county clinics—
it's all a blur.

Is all that supposed to have made me stronger?

Unemployment, off and on. TCOM, unemployment
compensation—food stamps...

Then, the other side....got a good raise. Got a new car. Moved
to 2 bedroom apt.

Now I'm looking for another place.

Good and bad are mixed.

That's life.

I can't dictate life. I can only face it. Lessons learned.

Am I better today?

Better than what?

Better than yesterday?

It's too early to tell.

I'll see how the day progresses.

Just keep breathing.

Keep putting one foot in front of the other.

Progress, not perfection.

Eat breakfast, shower, dress.

Even though it's an effort.

Today has much in it.

7/12/00

I'm a survivor.
And survivors must be smart.
There are degrees of intelligence—
"Street smarts"—
"Book smarts"—
I am both.
Some of my "street smarts" is really instinct.
Survival instinct. Protect yourself, Marilyn.
Until now, I've protected myself by avoiding pain.

191

Now I know I need to face it. Face the fears of abandonment. What others think—walk through the pain, end it, and then face life again.

Because now I know life is full of pain. And I have received my portion.

7/14/00

I'm in that fog again. Nothing seems real, like I'm in shock.

Shock over taking care of myself and getting out of that job gracefully. Before I cracked wide open.

I was pushed to the max, physically, mentally and emotionally.

I haven't cried in months. I've kept it all inside.

Also, I haven't been to Dr. Marsh since March.

If I were still working, I'd be in her office at least once a month.

So that ought to show that I'm much better off. Physically, at least, not working at that job.

I wonder. This no tears thing…Have I "hardened my heart"?

No more pretending I'm fine. I'm not fine.

I have lupus, diabetes, high blood pressure, hypothyroidism, and now this. I married badly. We divorced. I had two children to raise on my own. I married again and we divorced. I had to go to work. Did well until lupus reared its ugly head. I lost jobs. I quit dating.

Dad died.

Cat died.

My spirit died.

No wonder I'm depressed!

But I will get better.

7/16/00

I'm in an old familiar pattern. Going to move again. I'm straddling both here and there. Not much sense in doing much to this old place, except I can get rid of some stuff. Toss and organize.

Do I really need all this stuff? No.

7/17/00

Moving on my mind.
It all seems like too much trouble.
Damn this depression.
Clinical depression. Means chemical. So why don't I get some other kind
of help? Increase the Zoloft? Or try something else?
Damn headache. Earache. Even my knees ache a bit.
Pain is part of the depression.
Get rid of the depression.
I'm workin' on it!

7/21/00

I was supposed to be on jury duty. But I faxed them my doctor's excuse. I am sick, after all: diabetes, hypertension, hypothyroidism, and depression, not to mention my old friend lupus.

Wondering how much of a role ol' Lupe plays in this depression. Could be that's a major part. Add to that, the others —divorce, near poverty, jobs lost time after time…and this last one took the prize.

I know I should pray for "them." All those who crushed my spirit. I could not conform to Corporate America's policies. Most of the job was b.s. Very, very stressful to be micro-managed.

I wonder if this new person in my job has left yet.

I miss Sabbath terribly. I see her all around. I know her spirit is still here. Twenty years old. How old in cat years?

I feel free. Freedom means that you have nothing to prove, nothing to hide, and nothing to lose. Seems I've been trying to justify my existence all my life.

I don't need a reason to be here. God sent me here.

This damn depression is making me mad.

Yesterday, when I got to Macaroni Grill to meet Nancy and Joyce, Nancy said, "You sound depressed. What is it that's making you depressed?"

Well, I lost it! Said, "Hell if I know what's making me depressed. I wouldn't be depressed and seeing a counselor if I knew!"

Need to ask the support group about this. Will my irritation level get worse? Or am I just now being honest with others and myself?

About my snapping at others: Virgie said that's okay. I hear from her that I'm finally showing feelings. Even if they are misdirected.

Need to check this out with Dr. Wilson. I know he intends to get me to "crack" open and let my feelings out. He tried—subtly—but maybe he needs to take a "whack across the head" approach.

I know my little girl needed more than what she got. And I know I've been nurturing myself as best I can.

I know I'm still sick. Very sick indeed. About time I took a long vacation. I've been pushing very hard for over 10 years, without much of a break. Multiple events triggered this depression. So it's going to take a while to recover.

Car Wreck

My mind is a busy street.
Much traffic
Moving slowly,
Moving too fast.
Some cars stop at stoplights.
Is this where I am?
Waiting at a red light
For a green light?
The traffic in the other direction
Still streams by—
These are my unconscious thoughts
When I left work that last day
The cars collided at the intersection.

Tomorrow, I need to call Dr. Marsh for an appt. Re: meds. Find out about health ins.

Headache again.

Heavy heart feeling.

I cried a little yesterday, out of frustration.

How long, oh Lord, how long?

Now I know why people commit suicide. They are so hopeless and helpless.

I'm not there, but now I understand.

I hate this. Nothing is right, mentally, emotionally. I am drained. My eyes stare at nothing. Wide open but vacant.

Wish my counseling were going better.

"Fix me," I want to yell. "My spirit is broken." But only God can fix a broken spirit.

God, please fix my broken spirit.
Or tell me how I can mend it.
I'm Your child
And I'm hurting
Because—because.
Your child is ill, Lord.
Ill with a malady
That seems eternal,
Every day drags by.
No energy.
I know you want me to be happy.
And loving and giving
And using your gifts.
And I just can't do that right now.
Forgive me, Lord,
For my weaknesses.
I know they are not of Your work.
This must be teaching me a lesson
I need to learn.
Or many lessons.
I'm open and receptive
To Your voice, O Lord.
Speak to me
In a voice loud and clear—
What do You want of me?

7/24/00

Wrote and wrote, hoping I could cry. Nada. Zilch. Frozen.
Depression seems to linger.
Do I have CNS involvement?
Hell, aren't we all sick? One way or another.

7/26/00

Dealing with a lot of loss in my life. Well, DUH. But I've
never actually sat down and counted them up....
Loss of my father periodically.
Loss of roots with grandparents, etc.
Loss of my father when he went to Korea.
Loss of my father being at my 3rd grade play.
Loss of Whittier Elementary School in Lawton.
Loss of permanence.
Loss of control over my life as a brat.
Loss of leaving Linz...and grief.
Loss of friends.
Loss of first marriage...loss of the dream....
Loss of a second marriage...Ditto.
Loss of my home.
Loss of male relationships. Period.
Loss of health.
Loss of jobs, by choice or being let go.
Loss of income.
Loss of self-esteem, what I had of it.
Loss of my father to death.
Loss of Sabbath—my companion of 20 years.
And all of this is coupled with anger.

7/27/00

Virgie said yesterday that I'm a very strong woman. I have to agree.

I need to decide what to give Terri for her 40th birthday.

My diamond drop.

The reception is coming along just fine. Changed the hours to 5-7 p.m.

7/28/00

I have an appt. at 4 p.m. with Dr. Wilson.

Read him my stuff. Told him I hadn't had any emotions. Before, when I wrote it, or when I read it aloud. Just nothing. He said to keep writing about it.

Also told him about "why are you depressed?" And my response. He said that was progress.

The upshot of this session is that once again, I want the EVENT, not the PROCESS. It might take a couple of years to get well. And during that time, I need to take care of myself. Don't get into any relationships. I don't need the complication.

Besides, as sick as I am, I'd attract a sick one. Again.

I also realize all my life I've had losses and grief. And fear/anger that have never been resolved.

At the Global Nomads session of Overseas Brats, the leader had said, "*We all suffer from unresolved grief.*" That hit me right between the eyes.

7/29/00

About to get the condo. My realtor said one person who keeps promising a contract is on the way, but so far, nothing. So we'll get first dibs. Then if they don't take it, we'll offer $75,000.

Funny thing—How I was depressed most of the time I was with Hampton and nobody noticed. I put on a good front, I supposed. But my brain wasn't working right. No disguising that.

I haven't set foot inside an office since April 7. Soon it will be 4 months. I love it.

Working on issues. Re-read the Brats book. Work on my own book.

I put too much of my fantasies in the relationships I've had.

I overlooked the obvious because I didn't want to see the truth. I am now more aware of myself and of others.

I never trusted my intuition before. Now, I do.

I feel "leadened" today. Heavy legs that ache. Knees hurt, too.

Some days are gold, some days are lead.

Waiting for a gold day, darn it.

7/30/00

I'm getting the condo.

8/1/00

Got a message from my realtor. Miracles! The fax that the first buyer sent didn't all go through. So it's not binding.

The seller wants to close Aug. 25. That's the day Terri will be here!! And nobody knew that.

One more time I'm feeling sad to leave one place. Maybe this is a childhood memory. Moving again.

But this time it's in the same city. Even though it's a good move, I'm feeling the same feelings.

I know I have to get my childhood out of the way so I can heal.

There is no reality.

Only perception.

MY PERCEPTION IS:

I was, am, defective.

No, I'm not. I'm God's child.

God doesn't make defective products.

So I'm perfectly imperfect.

I'm impatient.

198

That's a truth.
I'm critical of myself.
I have to work.
Each day is a struggle.
But hey, life is difficult.
DYING IS THE EASY PART.
AND I'VE NEVER TAKEN THE EASY WAY OUT.
AND I NEVER WILL.

8/3/00

I'm seeing things out of the corner of my eyes. Depression can cause changes in vision.

Hmmm. I see things—differently.

I see reality…or my perception of reality changes.

I have "visions" of a new start.

Egad! How many times have I started over in my life?

Marriage #1, Divorce#1.

Started working.

Moved to FW.

Married #2.

Divorced #2.

Began working again.

Began dating again.

Began my recovery in Al-Anon.

Began my illness & recovery.

Began my depression.

Learned from it.

Began defining myself as a writer.

Right now, I write for personal satisfaction. I write because I have something to say. I write—because.

I write to glorify God who gave me a gift.

The little girl in me writes.

The teenager in me writes.

The hurt, happy, excited, depressed me writes.

I'm working on furniture placement in the new condo. Of course.

One of the first things to put up is my "Gruss Gott" plaque, by the front door.

8/6/00

I'm feeling better. Soon it will be 2 weeks since I started Celexa. It must be working.

Looked through some old pictures yesterday for Mom's reception. Cried over some.

8/8/00

Went to the condo for the inspection. Everything okay.

Still not feeling "normal." Up too late, slept too late—I feel I absolutely must have a nap in the afternoons. Thought I'd feel better by now. Give the Celexa more time.

Got my PTO check and one from Liberty Mutual for short-term disability. Funny thing how the ins. co. represents "liberty" to me. I've never really felt "liberty" before. I always felt I had to conform.

Now I don't have to obey anybody—except, of course, the law. But now I really feel like nobody can tell me what to do, when to do it and how.

God, I have always hated that. I have struggled against the "obey" part all my life—personally and professionally. It always went against my grain.

My spirit was being crushed at work. It wasn't just an idle thought. I felt it. And when I thought that I was too damn independent to do what my boss told me to do and how and when to do it, I rebelled. Inside, and told myself I was "bad" for rebelling.

The little girl stamped her foot (emotionally) and said NO. And was told to go to her room. The threat of being fired was a control tactic.

Well, for once in my life, I got my way.

And my way was OUT.

Out of the craziness, the rules, the chaos...out of there.

I don't need to punish myself for being me.
I don't need to punish myself for following my spirit.
It's time this little girl went out to play.

8/10/00

Call the movers today. Find pay schedule re: disability premiums for Cigna—THR. Appt. with Dr. Wilson at 4:00.

It really makes me angry when I try to think of something and I can't recall it...like the joke I read this morning..."Just a little melon collie." It takes me a while. Is this normal for my age? Is it part of the depression?

I find I'm still distancing myself from others. And that's sad.

8/11/00

Re-reading the book *Necessary Losses*. It is teaching me so much. I was in denial when I first read it, I'm sure. And I wasn't ready to "hear" what it had to teach me.

Packing. Calling utilities.

Work on Mom's program.

Set schedule for writing.

Discipline and routine are necessary.

8/12/00

Almost paralyzed this morning. Legs ache. Stiff.

I dreamed I was pulling yards and yards of stringy goo from my ear. Does that mean I haven't heard anything? Does it mean I'm now able to listen? My ear hurt last night before I went to bed. That's probably it.

8/15/00

Still having problems with sleep. Woke at 2:30 a.m. I just hate that.

HR called. Said I was anticipated to return to work July 7. Huh?

FMLA was from April to July.

Short-term disability was for 6 months. From July.

Then long-term kicks in.

I don't understand but when he asks if I want to extend it, I say yes.

10/4/00 Wednesday 10:30 p.m.

I moved here on 9/7/00. I am settled in my new townhouse. I feel a weight has fallen from me. And I have more room, and a courtyard and an office looking out onto the pool.

How did I get here?

I asked.

I took a chance on proposing this to Terri and she said yes.

How did I think of this? It had been rattling around in my head for a while. Just needed to get up my courage to ask…and then to look…and then to trust my instincts. So I got it and I moved.

I had almost too much help. "You've got too much stuff." I heard that so many times, it might be true. But I didn't get a chance to sort things out before I moved, so it had to come with me.

Besides, how much is "too much"? I think I'll be the judge of that.

Therapy is going well. Not sleeping well, though.

And right side of neck, head and right leg hurt. A lot.

Could be shingles path from before, re: my neck and head. The right leg is another matter. If not better soon, I need to see what's going on.

I seem to be searching for something.
I don't know what it is.
I don't need to buy anything, yet I shop. I just look. Antiques. Junk.
Resale. All just looking. Why?
Procrastination over writing? Maybe. Lord, help me. I hurt.
Physically, emotionally, spiritually. Show me what to do.

10/20/00 7:30 a.m.

Yesterday was a bitch. I had a meltdown about the insurance company
going to call. I missed another appointment with Philip. I'm sure he's pissed.
No excuse. Except I just feel I put down the wrong time. Again. Damn!
Another cognitive function gone south.

Can't do much reading for pleasure. Words don't make sense.
And forget math. It gets worse.

Can't quit obsessing over the disability crap. Choices are slim.
Flex time, Philip suggested, due to the sleep issues, wonder if he
said that because I missed the appt. yesterday?

Went to the dentist on Wed. Filling came out, I thought.
Wrong. It was some bonding crap that was turning loose. They
patched it again and did a temp. crown. To add to my financial
burden—$400—but I can pay it out. 3 mo. With no interest
under their credit card plan.

Damn. I hate being poor. I hate being old. I hate being sick. I hate
everything and everybody…almost. I'm just tired.

I get compulsive about the neatness of my house. Who's
coming? The Queen? I need to invite God into my day…all the
time.

10/20/00 — or 21?

I'm even confused about the date. I'm a wreck. A damn
shipwreck. I was sailing along with a comforting tide, enjoying the
breeze, when my ship hit the rocks. I'm drowning in a sea of self-
pity, doubt, insecurity, fear, and confusion. God, help me.

10/22/00 Sunday 8:30 a.m.

Feel like crap. Emotionally, I want to cry.

I'm tired of "depending on the charity of strangers," as they say. I wrestled with my budget yesterday. Till I was tired of it.

I'm at the age where I "should" be free to spend time with my grandchildren and travel and have a companion…and I have none of these.

My friends have money—I'm broke all the time.

I'm angry about that. And sad. Another loss to grieve.

Then what am I gonna do about it?

How can I make some money? Other than a 9-5 job?

Writing? Not now. I'm working on it. Feeling overwhelmed. Maybe I should just write articles and short stories.

Write a cover letter for my novels. Send out Sabbath's Room.

Go to a writer's group meeting.

10/23/00

Mom asked me, "What about your medical condition? What is it?" I took a deep breath and told her about the major depression. (Must remember to tell her it didn't start after I left work, but before.) She must think it's because I don't get out any —but I told her I do. Need to email her that fact. First, the acute stress disorder, then major depression. And that I've had it for a long time.

Just covered things up. For a long time. Put on a good front for everybody, including myself. Not authentic. Need to feel my feelings. More. And let them out.

Tough job. Never knew how to do that. Only felt anger, and lots of it. I'm still angry.

I'm angry that at my age, when I should be having a wonderful time with a retired, wonderful husband, traveling and doing whatever I want—that instead, I'm sick, broke and have nobody in my life. Nobody with me.

I'm angry that my friends have "more" than I do. That they go to places and do things I can't. Cruises? Gems, new furniture, etc. Indulging in their "wants" on a whim.

I'm angry that I married two men for the wrong reasons and they were the wrong men.

10/24/00 Tuesday 7:25 a.m.

Another bad night. Woke at 2 a.m. A dream woke me. Something about me trying to find the right key to lock a glass door. Frantic, because a "Mr. Smith" is trying to kill me. Terri is with me. With an axe.

Wrote it down. Must remember to tell Philip.

Then I'll go see the powers that be about my long-term disability. In a way, I'm glad I'm feeling and looking so bad. Then they'll know I'm really sick. I need that check. And others.

I can't possibly go back to work right now. There was a span in there where I felt pretty good. Was it the Celexa? This new Wellbutrin isn't helping. Must tell Dr. M. It also might take a couple of weeks?

I don't feel like writing or reading. Or going anywhere.

12/14/00 Thursday 9:45 a.m.

Where have I been? Haven't journaled in a couple of months.

Been to a real "shrink." Dr. Peter Kaminski. Started on Paxil. Seems to be working okay.

Was really "wigged out" on the Wellbutrin. Bawled and squalled in Fr. Bob's office...had a real "meltdown."

Also experienced a panic attack during a Bass Hall performance. (Go figure!) So I guess the Paxil takes some anxiety away.

Got my long-term disability from work approved! Good news. Must go on COBRA. Bad news is that it's $200 month. And they wanted 3 months all at once. Sent one month after conferring with Cigna. Must pay all by 1-31-01. Oh, well!

Must call Cigna for a refund of $90 I had to pay for the prescriptions.

205

Still semi-depressed? Anticipation over Christmas? Kept the kids last Sat. Joseph is such a character. Dad would have loved him. And Julia, too. Lord, help me to live long enough to see them grown.

1/6/2001 Saturday

Recovering from Christmas and all the activity. Saw Dr. Wilson Thurs. and Dr. Kaminski on Friday. Both say I'm doing fine. See Wilson next month; Kaminski in May.

I still have some issues to deal with. Always will. I find it difficult and irritating when bureaucracy gets in my way.

Incompetence. Cigna says I'm covered. Cigna says I'm not covered. Dr. Wilson hasn't been paid. Dr. K hates Cigna for the red tape. They are jeopardizing patient care. But they don't care.

Well, rant over.

1/9/01 Tuesday a.m.

Here I sit, in gown and robe
Listening to the birds singing
Squirrels dance on the roof.
No job to commute to.
No one to answer to.
Freedom, Liberty, Peace.
Truly grateful—I a.m.
For my disability.
God has seen fit
To use me in another way....
I wonder what it is.
Write about lupus
And depression
And recovery from both?
Or lead others
Out of the darkness
And into the light?

Perhaps both would be good.
What is holding me back?
Too many choices?
Divergent interests?
Am I being lazy?
Or taking care of myself?
I think writing
Six hours a day
Is not being lazy.
Writing is hard work.
Sometimes I ache from it.
Yet it's something
I must do.
God gave me the time
(After much complaining that I had no time)
And I hope He gave me talent, too.
With this time and talent, Lord,
I feel scattered and indecisive.
Please show me what to do next.
The writer's group on Wednesday
Should help me.
Fly in the direction of success.
They should provide a focus
So my limited energy is used best.
Go run my errands, mail my bills
Get stamps, pick up cleaning
And, oh, cash a check
And then I'm broke.
Is it too much to ask, Lord
To sell some of my work?
I'd love to travel
To writers' conferences.
Learn, and have fun, too.

1/10/01 Wednesday 7:45 a.m.

Found more pp of original brat story yesterday. Runs over 100 pp whereas my latest version is only about 86 pp. This longer version is no doubt from my old p.c. that crashed. So if I have any more useable stuff, I'll plug it in to my latest version.

Rewrite *Sabbath's Room* and send.

Finish brat story and send. Work on lupus story. Work on romance novel, *The Mall* and *The Wives*, as needed.

Send other short stories, articles.

Now I have a headache!

1/15/01 Monday 9:30 a.m.

I put out breadcrumbs
Which the birds ignore.
I set out a birdbath—
The birds prefer being dirty.
Lint from the dryer
Could build them a nest.
It sits untouched.
Birds not yet ready to mate.

1/16/01 Tuesday 9:45 a.m.

GraceWorks is my new business name.

Just popped into my head last night. By Grace, I am a writer. By Grace, I write.

1/26/01

Cleaned house. Went with Arlene to humane society and picked out a kitten. Four months old, black female, short hair. Looks like a baby Sabbath.

Can't pick her up till the 30th.

What name? Cleopatra. Cleo.

1/30/01

Picked up Cleo this morning She is already in charge. Took my place on the couch. She has been all over the house. Very quiet; and she followed me up and down the stairs. She helped me do laundry by sleeping on the pile of whites. Her jeweled collar is too big. I'll see if Bob can fix it tomorrow, when he comes for dinner.

2/6/01 6:30 p.m.

What a joy to have Cleo around. Tiny voice, but she makes her wishes known. She is banished from my bed at bedtime, since she wants to sleep, not with me, but on me.

And still wants to nurse. I can discourage her during the day, but when I'm asleep, it's impossible.

Will take her to the vet on Friday to have her stitches out.

Got a credit card in the mail yesterday. Only $350 limit, but that will do for Wichita in July. Send an email to Anne, Jane and Joyce to see who's going/share driving.

Need to register soon.

Need to finish my brat story. Take to Wichita? Or at least send it by email by then.

And lose 30 lbs by July? 20 would be okay, too.

Goals set. Tell Philip on Thurs.

2/13/01

Bought 6 prints on Saturday. Put them up in the study. All one huge wall of colorful prints. I like it. Also moved the large rug upstairs. Put it behind the bentwood rocker, w/3-drawer chest on it. Hung an ornate mirror over stand and put music boxes on display on it. Also put ornate gold mirror in downstairs bath with petit point pictures on either side. Also put all 4 of the Grevenburg watercolors in the bathroom. Looks great.

I know others might say I'm getting too much stuff, but I like it. I would have been right at home in a Victorian house. Eclectic, I'd say. I'm not decorating around a Japanese theme, even with the prints. No way. Too sparse.

And why do I feel like I must defend myself all the time? About anything? I have a right to do what I want as long as it doesn't interfere with anybody else.

I've always been on the defensive. Trying to explain myself. My actions, my feelings...me. As if I have to justify my existence.

I have a right to be here. I am a child of God, and He loves me. My existence is based on that premise. Not on anything else. If others judge me, it doesn't matter. If others hurt me, it doesn't matter.

That's about them, not me.

2/17/01

Going with Joyce and Nancy to the Kimbell. Then dinner.

Cleo is growing rapidly. Have had her for 18 days now. She's learned not to get up on the table or chairs. She wants to mess around on my office desk, but respects the water bottle squirt or just the sight of it will make her stop.

2/22/01

Need to complete my brat stuff by the time I leave for Wichita. Got some encouragement at writer's group last night. Linda supports my "italics" for the adult passages. I got beaten up pretty bad, I think. If I can take that, I can take rejection from an editor. It's about them, not my work.

Cleo is learning not to nurse on me. She has discovered the birds in the morning and is fascinated.

2/23/01

Not sleeping as well as I have been. Waking around 3 a.m. Last night, I woke at 12:30...after about an hour. Same pattern as before.

I'm going to the writers' conf. In Dallas. Get a chance to meet editors, publishers, agents and to "pitch" my brat book.

March-April

I broke my arm in Discovery Training in Dallas. Fell out of a chair, of all things. Had to leave the conference. Broke my "write" arm. DAMN!

5/3/01 Friday p.m.

Changed meds again. Dr. K. said Effexor, 150 mg. Is what I need now. Tapering off the Paxil. Also got another sleep prescription.

Damn! The broken arm sent me into another downward spiral. Increased Paxil—didn't help. I just was back in the pit. No energy. No joy. Didn't want to go anywhere. Can't write.

My "raison d'etre" was taken from me. Suffered from the criticism at Writers' Roundtable Conference in March.

And Philip said that's where the newer depression began.

Damn.

Today—I'm straightening out drawers, under the sink, etc. Will tackle the office next. Oh, migod, what a job.

Just do it in little pieces.

5/6/01 Saturday

Qu'elle surprise! Mom called this morning. Usual small talk between us. Then I asked her if "the family ever had anybody like a crazy old aunt locked up in the attic. I mean, did anybody suffer a clinical depression, like me?"

She said, "Well, when your Grandpa Garrett died, I lost a whole lot of weight, remember? I was skin and bones and everything seemed to stick in my throat. So I went to the doctor, finally, and he told me I was clinically depressed and put me on something—I don't remember what—but I got better."

Shazaam! Wait till I tell Philip Wilson this latest.

There's more to it than what she told me, too. Consider this that I already knew:

Her mother died when she was three.

Her father left her with her mother's family on the Indian Reservation at Ajo, AZ.

The Richardsons—Emily's father, Tom, was married to an Indian (name unknown).

The Richardsons, according to Mom, kept her in the same dress, day after day, until it literally fell apart. Then they'd buy her another dress. She was also encouraged to eat all the candy she wanted.

(To this day, she loves to shop for new clothes and her candy dish is always full.)

Grandpa Garrett went off to Denver and met and married Fern Herrmann. She was a large, stern, no-nonsense German-descent woman. According to my mother, Fern took one look at the house on the reservation, with no screens on the windows, little more than adobe huts, and put her foot down. She would not live there. GP got another job with So. Pacific RR and they moved.

When I was born, I was the family baby. Spoiled? Nah.

5/7/01

Need to write. Arm still hurts, though.
DAMN!

Philip Wilson told me this would be a rough time…between meds. Between depression and recovery. "Between the devil and the deep blue sea."

212

Feel like shit.
When will I feel "normal"?
Am *I* the crazy old aunt in the attic?

5/10/01 2 p.m.

Had a meltdown awhile ago. Assholes at Liberty Mutual denied me my check. No deposit to my account, yet.

I called the powers that be at my former job. They will be checking and will call them.

I left a message for Ms. G to call me.

I called Philip Wilson and left a message. Whine.

6/7/01 Thursday p.m.

Another day with no check. No word. I should be freaking out. Instead, I'm just pissed.

God, why must I wait? You know my needs.

I need to pay my bills.

Please let me know soon. I trust You. I know You know better than I.

It's just so very hard to trust.

7/3/2001

I wake this morning, fix coffee, take out the trash, check my email and fix breakfast.

All of a sudden, sobs break out.

I am so tired of all this crap! I cry and eat breakfast. Call the AC repairman to check the freon.

I feel so adrift.

Losing my balance often now. Am I over-medicated?

But it began in March. Before all these new meds.

Of course, I'm thinking, "Brain tumor."

7/6/01 Friday

Crying. For no apparent reason. Other than I am so tired of the crap with the insurance company and I have no money again...still....

God, tell me. Loud and clear. What do I need to do?

I am willing to go back to work if need be.

10/19/01

Much has happened.

Too much.

September 11. Oh, God.

Doug's death.

My going on his Social Security—and I had already checked on drawing my own benefits the week before he died. So all was in place and I got my check that same month. While it's not going to cover all my expenses, it will take care of the essentials. Perhaps that was the reason I managed to stay married to him over 10 years. God knew what I needed, more than I could have imagined.

Take trip to Alpine/Toronto, with my mother's family, to explore the grounds where I was born.

Must write about Doug's death. Have I done that? Probably not. I'm sad that he had to die to find peace. It was a terrible death from cancer. Lauri is taking it very hard. I wish I had closure. Could see her more often—but only by being "here" for her, can I help. She must know that she'll always have me.

The Twin Tower/Pentagon attacks seemed unreal. I also haven't worked since then. Many others are out of work, for real. I asked the temporary agency for more work. So far, an offer of temp to perm, but I can't do that. And, oh, yeah, I'm being published!

214

Here Endeth the Journal

Today, I'm okay.

Not "cured," but better

Gradually, year by year, I have been recovering. I've had two books published and moved again. I know lupus will never be entirely defeated. At best, I can arrange a peaceful coexistence with this wild gypsy Lupe who runs about setting smoldering campfires in various parts of my body.

I expect that some day I will have another flare, but so far so good. If I can manage my stressors, get enough rest, follow doctors' suggestions, I'll continue to do well—and try to help others through the Lupus Foundation of America.

Today, lupus is in a coma. My focus has shifted from SLE to managing my diabetes, which has sprung into life again. To quote Roseanne Roseannadanna: "It's always something."

I discovered some things along the way, one of which was I had been taking the same action, expecting different results, as far as my working career was concerned.

When I got my divorce, all I could do was type, so I became a secretary. While I was a darn good secretary, this was not my "calling," and at my last place of employment, I vowed that I would not spend the rest of my life working to make somebody else rich, adhering to arbitrary rules and procedures—in short, I would find work that meant something to me, personally, that my soul had been seeking.

You can call that impractical, but to me, it's part of what had made me ill in the first place.

That inner voice that kept telling me I was in the wrong marriage, the wrong job—but fear had kept me from taking action.

After facing lupus, I felt I had no fear left.

To paraphrase Pogo, "I have seen the enemy and it is me."

Most of the time, lupus is far from my mind.

And always, always, I pray that I never forget what this disease has taught me.

215

To be patient with others;
To be humble before God and my fellow man;
To be compassionate with those less fortunate;
To treasure every moment of every day;
To stay in The Now;
To know that in the end, it's just me and God.

Marilyn Celeste Morris
Fort Worth, Texas
November 2004